"Sleep is one of the few universals of life, and yet we still know little about it. In particular, the reasons we don't sleep can be as mystifying as the reasons we do. *The Insomnia Workbook* is a comprehensive, scholarly, and clearly written review of what we know about the architecture of sleep, how insomnia disrupts that architecture, and what can be done to rebuild a healthy sleep pattern."

—Robert McGrath, Ph.D., director of the Ph.D. program in clinical psychology and director of the MS Program in clinical psychopharmacology at Fairleigh Dickinson University in Teaneck, NJ

"Silberman has distinguished herself in the diagnosis and treatment of sleep disorders. There are still far too few dedicated sleep professionals available. Her new book is needed to promote greater understanding of why insomnia is far and away the most common manifestation of underlying sleep disorder and what to do to relieve this distressing condition."

—Bruce Nolan, MD, FACP, FAASM, sleep center medical director at Miller School of Medicine, University of Miami

"Silberman has taken the difficult topic of insomnia and provided an informative review not only of normal sleep, but also of common sleep problems. She discusses treatments for people having difficulty falling asleep and staying asleep using up-to-date medical and psychological treatments. The book is sure to be of interest to people with trouble sleeping and readers who simply wish to learn more about the fascinating world of sleep."

—Glenn R. Singer, MD, I sleep disorder centers at Broward General Medic auderdale, FL

"The idea of a comprehensive insomnia workbook, starting from the basics of sleep to diagnosis and management, is brilliant. This book is up-to-date and serves as an 'all you need to know about sleep' guide. It is easy to read and understand, keeps the reader's attention, and acts like a teaching aid. I would recommend this book to anyone interested in learning about the various intricacies of sleep, and to any professional who requires in-depth information. Silberman has further enriched the world of sleep with her contribution."

—Vipin Garg, MD, FCCP, FAASM, director of the sleep disorders center at Trinitas Hospital in Elizabeth, NJ, and assistant professor of medicine at Seton Hall University

the insomnia workbook

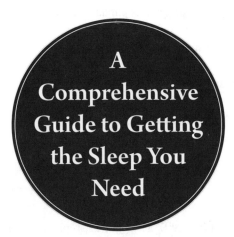

A Comprehensive Guide to Getting the Sleep You Need

STEPHANIE A. SILBERMAN, PH.D., DABSM

New Harbinger Publications, Inc.

Distributed in Canada by Raincoast Books

Copyright © 2008 by Stephanie A. Silberman
New Harbinger Publications, Inc.
5674 Shattuck Avenue
Oakland, CA 94609
www.newharbinger.com

Epworth Sleepiness Scale (ESS), © 1990-1997 M.W. Johns, reprinted here with permission of M.W. Johns.

DBAS-16, © 2007 Charles M. Morin, reprinted here with permission of Charles M. Morin.

All Rights Reserved
Printed in the United States of America

Acquired by Jess O'Brien; Cover design by Amy Shoup;
Edited by Jasmine Star

Library of Congress Cataloging-in-Publication Data on file with the publisher

FSC
Mixed Sources
Product group from well-managed
forests and other controlled sources

Cert no. SW-COC-002283
www.fsc.org
© 1996 Forest Stewardship Council

11 10 09

10 9 8 7 6 5 4 3 2 1   First printing

This book is dedicated to my husband, Dr. Frank Hull, who encouraged and inspired me to write this book. His own expertise in the area of sleep medicine, along with his passion and dedication to the field, is truly admirable. And to my son, Elliot, for his love, kisses, and many hugs.

Contents

Acknowledgments vii

Foreword ix

Introduction 1

CHAPTER 1
The Basics About Sleep 5

CHAPTER 2
What Is Insomnia? 19

CHAPTER 3
Medications for Insomnia 45

CHAPTER 4
Sleep Hygiene 61

CHAPTER 5
Relaxation Techniques 75

CHAPTER 6
Sleep Logs 89

CHAPTER 7
Stimulus Control and Sleep Restriction 105

CHAPTER 8
Controlling Anxiety and Irrational Thoughts 119

CHAPTER 9
Managing Daytime Stress and Maintaining a Healthy Lifestyle 145

CHAPTER 10
Preventing Relapse 157

CHAPTER 11
Parasomnias 163

CHAPTER 12
Women and Sleep. 169

Resources 177

References 179

Acknowledgments

To family and friends who encouraged me throughout this project, thank you for sharing your time and lending your support.

Thank you to my acquisitions editor at New Harbinger Publications, Jess O'Brien, for his belief in the value of this book from the beginning, and for helping it come to fruition. Excellent feedback from editors Jess Beebe and Jasmine Star helped to improve the final manuscript.

A special thanks to my parents, Myron and Dr. Teresa Silberman, for showing me the value of education, hard work, kindness, and compassion to others.

Foreword

Almost everyone has experienced an occasional poor night's sleep due to worries, an impending deadline, or a sick child. For at least 10 percent of the adult population, though, insomnia is a chronic and burdensome problem. It is also the most prevalent of all sleep disorders. Although there is a tendency to trivialize or make fun of sleep problems, chronic difficulty sleeping produces daytime fatigue, mood disturbances, and problems with attention and concentration, and it often makes otherwise simple tasks difficult to accomplish. When left untreated, insomnia increases absenteeism from work and heightens the risk of depression.

While there is no doubt that insomnia should be taken seriously, people with sleep problems are ⟨n⟩ discouraged by the lack of resources available to treat the problem. Of course, we are inundated ⟨ad⟩vertisements for various sleeping pills. Although they may be useful in the short term under some ⟨circums⟩tances, there are risks of habituation and dependency associated with their long-term usage. ⟨Over-the⟩-counter medications and natural products, as well as alcohol, should be avoided altogether, ⟨ther⟩e is no evidence that they work, and they are not without risks. So, what are the treatment ⟨op⟩t for those with chronic insomnia?

⟨In th⟩is workbook, Dr. Silberman eloquently describes an effective self-help program for overcoming ⟨b⟩ased on psychological and behavioral principles. Indeed, there is now solid scientific evidence ⟨cogniti⟩ve behavioral therapy is an effective treatment alternative—if not the treatment of choice— ⟨for⟩ insomnia. In addition to being safer and often more acceptable to patients, this approach ⟨lo⟩nger lasting results than sleep medication. Nonetheless, it remains underutilized by health ⟨provide⟩rs and is not always readily accessible to those who need it most. The number of sleep clinics ⟨grew⟩ tremendously over the past several years, but, unfortunately, few sleep professionals have ⟨been⟩ offering specialized cognitive behavioral therapy for insomnia.

⟨The I⟩nsomnia Workbook fills an important gap and is a welcome addition to the self-help books ⟨I⟩t provides a step-by-step approach that includes all of the major therapeutic components that ⟨are⟩ shown effective in the management of insomnia around the world. These methods include ⟨behavioral⟩ approaches aimed at changing poor sleep habits, psychological methods targeting unhelpful beliefs and thinking patterns that often fuel the vicious cycle of insomnia, and practical information for maintaining healthy sleep practices. Relaxation techniques and other stress management methods are offered to address daytime stressors and unhealthy lifestyles that contribute to nighttime sleep difficulties. This book also provides useful information about sleep medications and practical guidelines for discontinuing them. Several self-assessment tools—including a sleep journal, questionnaires and checklists, and practical homework assignments—make this workbook a very accessible and user-friendly resource. This manual also provides some basic facts about normal sleep and about sleep disorders other than insomnia, including nightmares, sleepwalking and sleep terrors, sleep-related eating disorder, and women's sleep issues connected to premenstrual syndrome, pregnancy, and menopause.

The Insomnia Workbook will be an invaluable resource for anyone with sleep difficulties, and for therapists treating them. It can be used as a self-help manual or as a companion workbook to therapist-guided treatment. This practical and evidence-based manual gives hope of relief to those millions of people who suffer from insomnia by itself or in association with other psychological or medical conditions such as anxiety, depression, or chronic pain.

Charles M. Morin, Ph.D.
Professor of Psychology
Director, Sleep Disorders Center
Université Laval, Québec, Canada
Canada Research Chair on Sleep Disorders

Introduction

"I'm sitting in front of the television at night, feeling so tired that I can barely keep my eyes open. But the moment my head hits the pillow, I'm wide awake!" —Brett

"I don't know what's wrong with me. I don't feel all that stressed during the day, but when I lie in bed at night, all I can think about are the millions of things I need to do tomorrow at work, at home, with my kids…my mind just won't shut off." —Lori

"I fall asleep fine at the beginning of the night, but then I wake up around 3 or 4 a.m. and cannot fall back asleep. I'm not sure what wakes me up. Sometimes I have to go the bathroom, but I don't think that's it. I just lie in bed, staring at the clock, wondering why I can't sleep straight through the night like my husband lying next to me!" —Suzanne

"I'm just not tired when I get into bed. I don't know what's wrong with me. I used to sleep seven to eight hours per night and never had a problem. But ever since my son was born, I have problems falling asleep and staying asleep. It's aggravating, because I need my energy during the day in order to be productive." —Beth

"My wife says that it started after I changed jobs, and maybe she's right. I'm really not sure, but all I know is that I wake up in the middle of the night with my heart pounding, have trouble breathing, and then feel angry that I can't fall back asleep. I've been to my doctor and a specialist, and there's nothing wrong with my heart. I don't know why I get so worked up, but it needs to stop!" —Dave

"I've taken nearly every sleeping pill you can imagine. They all seem to work fine at first, but after a couple f weeks, I'm back to where I started: trouble falling asleep for hours on end, and then once I do fall asleep, I ake up after one or two hours. Why don't these medications work better for me?" —Karen

don't feel depressed, and I don't think I'm anxious. I just don't understand why I can't sleep. I lie in bed at ht thinking about how long it will take me to fall asleep. There's nothing else on my mind, but the hours are t ticking away." —Chris

Do these words sound familiar to you? If so, you're not alone. Recent research indicates that nearly one-third of Americans suffer from insomnia at some point during their lives (Ohayon 2002). Although it may feel frustrating to be one of those people, take heart: Effective treatment that doesn't involve medications is available to you, here, within these pages. This workbook is designed to help you overcome your insomnia at home, in a step-by-step approach that involves your active participation. You will need to devote time to reading this book thoroughly, filling out the questionnaires, and doing the exercises and other activities recommended, all of which will help you achieve a successful night's sleep.

There are different types of insomnia, including trouble falling asleep, trouble staying asleep, and early morning awakenings. Insomnia can be short term, lasting from a few days to a few weeks. It can also be chronic, lasting months or even years on end. The severity of insomnia can also vary, from occasional bad nights that occur once or twice per week to significant problems sleeping five to seven nights per week. Insomnia can mean waking up once each night or several times per night and having trouble falling back asleep, or it can mean lying in bed trying to fall asleep for thirty minutes or three hours. In other words, insomnia can vary from person to person. And even if you don't have insomnia, you may not be completely satisfied with your sleep and may be interested in improving it. If so, you too will find this book helpful. The techniques in this book can help anyone sleep more soundly.

Like most things, overcoming insomnia doesn't just happen overnight. But if you stick with the suggestions and guidelines in this book, you should start sleeping better soon. Depending on what the root cause of your sleep problem is, it may take anywhere from a few days to several weeks before you see positive changes in your sleep patterns. The most important thing is not to give up in the early stages. Give your mind and body a chance to overcome insomnia in a way that doesn't rely on medications, herbs, or supplements by using the cognitive behavioral methods outlined in this workbook.

Cognitive behavioral therapy is a type of psychological treatment that focuses on behaviors and ways of thinking and the role that they play in creating and maintaining certain patterns in a person's life. When these patterns are maladaptive, they cause problems. The key is to identify and change the problematic behaviors and thoughts. The sleep program in this book includes both behavioral and cognitive aspects, with specific chapters focusing on various behaviors and thoughts that may be contributing to your sleep problem and offering techniques to modify or change them. Behavioral approaches include improving your sleep hygiene (chapter 4), practicing relaxation techniques (chapter 5), using sleep logs (chapter 6), and implementing stimulus control and sleep restriction (chapter 7). The primary cognitive approach involves controlling anxiety and irrational thoughts (chapter 8). Chapter 9 discusses both behavioral and cognitive techniques for managing daytime stress and maintaining a healthy lifestyle.

HOW THIS BOOK IS ORGANIZED

This workbook offers a hands-on approach to the treatment of insomnia. You may not have a sleep specialist available to you where you live, or you may not have the time or resources to see a specialist in person. For that reason, this workbook is intended to replicate the experience of working with an insomnia sleep specialist, from the initial consultation and assessment of the nature of your sleep problem t instruction in cognitive behavioral approaches and other techniques for improving your sleep. There w be questionnaires and activities for you to do along the way. These are the same types of questions a approaches that a sleep specialist would use in face-to-face appointments. Using this workbook, you can take charge of improving your sleep.

To give you a better idea of what to expect as you work through this book, here's a breakdown of the chapters and what they'll include. Chapter 1 discusses the fundamentals of sleep, with information on typical sleep patterns, sleep in different stages of life, the effects of sleep deprivation, and common myths about sleep. Chapter 2 describes the different types of insomnia, including common psychological and medical causes, and other sleep disorders that may be affecting your ability to sleep. It also discusses sleep and aging. Because sleeping medications are so widely used but also so potentially problematic, chapter 3 provides information on medications for insomnia, including over-the-counter drugs, herbal remedies, and prescription sleeping pills. It discusses how sleeping aids may be causing problems for you, and when and how to safely stop taking sleeping medications.

The treatment portion of the book begins in chapter 4, with a review of sleep hygiene and important ways to change some of your behaviors so that they help promote sleep. Chapter 5 emphasizes the importance of relaxation and describes specific relaxation techniques that you can learn and practice. Chapter 6 explains sleep logs and how to use them to record data about your sleep. The information you gather is important, and you'll use it as you continue working through the book. Chapter 7 explains stimulus control and sleep restriction. These techniques are a key part of the approach in this book. They can be used to alter your sleep patterns, and chapter 7 will explain exactly how to do this. Chapter 8 moves on to cognitive factors that may be making your sleep worse and provides you with ways to control any anxiety and irrational thought processes that may be interfering with your sleep. Chapter 9 will help you manage daily stress and maintain a healthy lifestyle. Beyond helping improve your sleep, this will enhance your overall well-being. The final treatment chapter (chapter 10) is devoted to preventing relapse and offers tips on how to handle an occasional bad night.

The two remaining chapters cover other areas of interest in the realm of sleep. Chapter 11 describes parasomnias, or abnormal behaviors during sleep. These include sleepwalking, sleep terrors (also called night terrors), confusional arousals, sleep-related eating disorder, REM sleep behavior disorder, and nightmare disorder. Chapter 12 focuses on issues that may affect women's sleep, such as PMS, pregnancy, and menopause. Lastly, there is a resources section with useful websites and places to buy relaxation CDs.

WHO I AM AND WHY I WROTE THIS BOOK

You may be wondering why I decided to write a workbook on insomnia. Since I first started working in the field of sleep medicine, I've been amazed at how many people have trouble sleeping. Everywhere I go, people ask me questions about sleep. Some of the most frequent questions include "How many hours of sleep do I need each night?" "What's causing me to toss and turn for an hour while I'm trying to fall asleep?" "Can napping during the day affect my sleep at night?" "Why do I feel wide awake when I get into bed each night, and why I am waking up during the night?"

With insomnia being such a widespread problem, I decided to write a self-help book on insomnia in a workbook format to answer some of these questions and provide solutions for difficulties with sleeping. The workbook format allows you, the reader, to actively participate in learning about and improving your sleep rather than just passively turning the pages.

I am a licensed clinical psychologist and board-certified sleep medicine specialist, but I'm also a working mother, wife, and activist in my community. I'm the type of person who loves to be busy, but I also know the importance of slowing down and simply enjoying life. I know how hard it can be to achieve and maintain that "perfect balance" in your life—the kind of balance that allows you to feel fulfilled in your work and daily activities and to also feel calm and at peace with the world around you. This book is a way for me to use my experience and expertise to help people with one of the most vital and important things we do every day: sleep—and sleep well so that we can maintain happy, healthy lives.

CHAPTER 1

The Basics About Sleep

Before getting into the evaluation and treatment of insomnia, it's important to have an understanding of the basic processes underlying sleep. In other words, what is normal sleep? This means having a discussion on the stages of sleep and *sleep architecture*, meaning the cycling in and out of the different stages of sleep during the night. Sleep architecture is a way of quantifying the amount and percentage of time spent in each stage of sleep. It changes from night to night, depending on both internal and external factors. For example, snoring or sleep-disordered breathing is an internal factor that can affect sleep architecture. External factors such as drinking alcohol, taking certain medications, or ambient noise can also alter sleep architecture. When evaluating sleep, other factors are considered, such as the number of times a person wakes up in the night and the length of those awakenings, how long it takes to fall asleep, and what percentage of the time spent lying in bed is actually spent sleeping.

THE STAGES OF SLEEP AND THE SLEEP CYCLE

Sleep is divided into different stages, each associated with different types of brain waves. If someone were to place electrodes on your head to measure your brain's electrical activity as you slept, they would be able to determine the frequency of your brain waves and, therefore, when you were in particular stages of sleep. This measurement of electrical activity, called *electroencephalography*, or EEG, led to the discovery of the various stages of sleep. The following discussion of the various sleep stages will help you understand what is considered to be normal brain wave activity during sleep.

As of 2007, the guidelines of the American Academy of Sleep Medicine classify sleep into four stages: stage N1, stage N2, stage N3, and stage R sleep (Iber et al. 2007). The first three stages are part of NREM (pronounced non-rem) sleep.

Stage N1

Stage N1 (NREM1), formerly known as stage 1 sleep, occurs when you're first falling asleep. It's the lightest stage of sleep, and is really the transition between wakefulness and sleep. During this stage, you may have slow, rolling eye movements as you begin to lose conscious awareness of your environment. Due to how light this stage is, you can still be easily awakened by external stimuli. You may also experience muscle twitches or jerks. The average young adult sleeper doesn't spend much time in stage N1 sleep. It usually accounts for less than 10 percent of total sleep time.

Stage N2

Next is stage N2 (NREM2), previously called stage 2 sleep. This stage of sleep is a bit deeper than stage N1 and is distinguished on an EEG by sleep spindles and K-complexes. A *sleep spindle* is a burst of 12- to 16-hertz waves that occur during stage N2 sleep. A *K-complex* is a waveform with a brief high-voltage peak that occurs randomly during stage N2 sleep, but can also occur in response to auditory stimuli in the sleeping environment. During this stage, conscious awareness of the external environment disappears and there is decreased muscle activity. Depending on your age, you're likely to spend between 35 and 55 percent of your time in stage N2 sleep on an average night (Bowman and Mohsenin 2003). In other words, you spend the most time in stage N2 sleep.

Stage N3

Next is stage N3 sleep, which was previously referred to as stages 3 and 4 sleep. Also known as slow-wave sleep or delta sleep, stage N3 sleep is defined by slow-wave activity, or delta waves, on an EEG. Slow-wave sleep is thought to be the most restorative part of the sleep cycle; it's also the deepest period of sleep and the most difficult time to wake a person up. Most slow-wave sleep occurs in the first third of the night, with significantly less or even no slow-wave sleep occurring later in the night. You may recall instances where someone said that you answered the phone or had a brief conversation with them after you had fallen asleep, but you don't remember it. If you were woken up from slow-wave sleep, you would probably have little or no recollection of it in the morning. Young adults spend between 13 and 23 percent of their sleep cycle in delta sleep, but that decreases to 5 to 18 percent with age (Bowman and Mohsenin 2003). This decrease may, in fact, just be part of aging, although some sleep researchers believe that it has more to do with how we assess sleep stages and greater difficulty in detecting delta sleep in older people. Sleep disorders such as sleepwalking, sleeptalking, sleep terrors (also called night terrors), and bed-wetting usually occur during delta sleep. *Confusional arousals*, which are episodes of considerable confusion during and after arousal from sleep, also generally occur during delta sleep. (Most of these sleep disorders, known as *parasomnias*, are discussed in chapter 11.)

Stage R

Next is stage R sleep, also known as stage REM sleep. REM stands for rapid eye movement. Most people think of this as the time when dreaming takes place, and although most dreaming does occur during stage REM sleep, it can also occur in other stages. REM sleep differs from slow-wave sleep in that it's the most active period of sleep for your brain, and for certain physiologic responses in your body, such as breathing, heart rate, and temperature regulation. It's also much lighter, which is why it's easier to wake up from REM sleep. When you wake up directly from stage REM sleep, you have a higher chance of remembering your dreams. We spend about 20 to 25 percent of our sleep time in stage REM sleep as young adults, and about 15 to 20 percent as we get older (Bowman and Mohsenin 2003). During REM sleep, your muscles relax to a point of near paralysis. This is normal during REM sleep, because it stops you from acting out your dreams. Some people have a sleep disorder called REM sleep behavior disorder (RBD), in which the muscle paralysis during REM malfunctions, so they move during their dreams. However, that isn't what's supposed to happen during normal sleep.

The Sleep Cycle

Progressing through the different stages of sleep outlined above is a *sleep cycle*. On a typical night, a person goes through several sleep cycles, although usually not through stage N1 again unless the person has woken up during the night or has frequent arousals due to a sleep disorder such as sleep apnea. Each cycle typically lasts from 90 to 110 minutes. Depending on how long you sleep, you may have four or five sleep cycles each night.

SLEEP CHANGES DURING THE LIFE SPAN

The way we sleep changes significantly during infancy and childhood and then remains relatively stable during adulthood. The number of hours infants and young children sleep per day is very high and slowly decreases until adolescence or early adulthood. Similarly, there are big differences in sleep architecture between newborns, young children, older children, and adolescents or adults. For example, children tend to spend much more time in delta sleep than adults. Since the brain isn't fully developed in babies and very young children, their brain waves look different from an adult's. From around age three through adulthood, the percentage of REM remains the same, at about 20 to 25 percent of the sleep period. In most people, however, REM sleep decreases further after about age fifty. In addition, some sleep behaviors that are considered normal during childhood may cause problems in adults. These include sleepwalking, sleep terrors, and confusional arousals, which will be discussed in chapter 11, on parasomnias.

Infancy and Childhood

Babies who only fall asleep while nursing or drinking a bottle have a harder time falling asleep on their own. If they're used to falling asleep in a parent's arms, while drinking, then they won't want to fall asleep in other circumstances. But babies need practice falling asleep on their own. Once they learn that they're able to do it, everyone's life will be easier at bedtime.

The same is true for children who push the limits when it's time to go to bed, asking for one more glass of milk or water, one more bedtime story, one more tuck into bed, or one more hug and kiss. Although you may find yourself giving in to these demands in the hopes that this will help your child get to sleep, caving in is likely to make the situation worse. Children need limits throughout the day, and especially at bedtime, otherwise they'll continue to push the limits further and further. In addition, giving in to these demands can set the stage for your child to develop a sleep problem, as your child begins to believe it's only possible to fall asleep under certain conditions.

Some children have fears at bedtime. They may be nervous that you won't be there when they wake up, or be scared that there are monsters hiding in the closet or under the bed. Children can also get upset when they think they might be missing out on something fun while they're sleeping. Reassure your child that everyone sleeps, including you, and that sleep is an important part of life. You can teach your child about good sleep hygiene (covered in chapter 4) from an early age and emphasize that we need sleep in order to grow big and strong and to feel good during the day. Children learn by example, so if they see you preparing for bed, they may want to do so themselves. Even if you aren't going to bed at the same time, you can still set the mood and tone by brushing your teeth together, dimming the lights, and having everyone get ready for bed as a family.

Adolescence and Early Adulthood

A variety of factors can affect sleep during the teenage years and early adulthood. People in this age group often stay up late to go to parties, to hang out with their friends, to study or do homework, or for a variety of other reasons. It's common for them to go to bed later and have trouble waking up on time. With schools starting at such an early hour, this can mean teenagers (and some college students) are very tired during the day, especially in the morning hours. They may sleep much later on the weekends, showing that their bodies do indeed need more sleep than they're getting.

Though it may seem far-fetched, it's important for people in this age group to maintain a regular sleep schedule. Although there may be a natural tendency to go to sleep later and wake up later, this schedule doesn't fit particularly well with our society, which places academic or occupational demands on us in the mornings. Plus, staying up late (and getting up late) can develop into delayed sleep phase syndrome. (This disorder is discussed in chapter 2, and treatment recommendations are given in chapter 4.)

Parenting

Although welcoming a new baby into the world is a joyful occasion, it also marks the start of serious sleep deprivation. Newborns wake up often during the night, sometimes as much as every one to two hours. If you're lucky, your baby may sleep for longer stretches, like three to four hours, but don't count on it at the beginning. Babies usually wake up to nurse or have a bottle, both of which require active involvement of a parent or caregiver. For mothers, nursing is a beautiful, special time between you and your baby—but also an exhausting time. People often say that mothers should nap when the baby naps, but that can be hard to do. And for either parent, the endless tasks and responsibilities that come with parenthood mean you might find it hard to squeeze in a shower, let alone a nap. However, taking care of yourself is important, so having a nap when you can isn't a bad idea if you're feeling very tired.

Even once your baby is sleeping for longer periods during the night, it still may be only a five- to six-hour stretch. Unless you go to bed at the exact same time as your baby, it's likely that you'll still be missing out on precious hours of sleep each night. You may also find yourself checking on your baby during the night, which can cut into your sleep. And what about when your child is sick at night? That's an obvious time when parents lose sleep.

Sleep terrors are quite common in young children. They result in a blood-curdling scream when the child is terrified by frightening images, but the child is often unable to recall anything about it the next morning. Still, your child's sleep terrors are likely to disturb your sleep. Not only can they make it hard to settle your child down, it may be hard for you to fall back asleep after such an upsetting disruption. If your child experiences any other parasomnias that occur during the night, such as sleepwalking or confusional arousals, this can also disrupt your sleep. (See chapter 11 for more on parasomnias.) Some children also wet their beds. If this is the case, you may find yourself changing sheets in the middle of the night, helping your child change into clean pajamas, and so on. All of this means less sleep for you.

Sleep and Aging

As you'll learn in chapter 2, insomnia can be related to an underlying medical or psychological disorder, and as we get older, medical conditions become more common, as does taking medications for those conditions. No matter what your age, it's important to figure out whether your sleep problems are related to a medical problem or to medication side effects, but this is particularly true if you're over the age of fifty-five.

In addition, lifestyle changes such as retirement can lead to increased sleep problems. If you're used to a set daily schedule, with many duties and responsibilities at the workplace and at home, it would seem that retirement holds the promise of being a relaxing, peaceful time. However, without a set schedule, some retirees find themselves sleeping during the day, being more sedentary (for example, maybe watching a lot of TV), and not maintaining a regular bedtime and wake time. All of these issues can lead to sleep problems. In addition, retirement can bring certain stressors, including living on a fixed income, dealing with boredom and a feeling of being unproductive, or moving to another part of the country and losing your social support network.

A particularly difficult issue with regard to aging is that it can be hard to watch friends and loved ones, especially your spouse, develop health problems and, at some point, die. Many people complain that getting older is depressing, particularly because of health issues and, for some, a more limited sphere of daytime activities compared to earlier in life. For some people retirement may be a time of enjoyment, with the freedom to travel, try new activities, and spend more time with family members, but for others it's a stressful phase of life that can lead to sleepless nights.

SLEEP DEPRIVATION

Now that you've had a glimpse of the many changes that take place across the life span with regard to sleep needs, sleep architecture, and certain sleep-related behaviors, let's talk about what happens to your body when you don't get enough sleep.

A U.S. Centers for Disease Control and Prevention (CDC) study released in February 2008 estimated that about 10 percent of U.S. adults don't get enough sleep each night. In fact, as many as 38 percent of people surveyed felt that they didn't get a sufficient amount of sleep for seven or more days during the month. In addition, the study concluded that around 50 to 70 million American adults are chronically sleep deprived, due to either sleep disorders, lifestyle, or occupational factors (Atkins 2008). Not everyone experiences sleep deprivation, or not getting enough sleep, the same way. For example, your mood may be affected, which can lead to symptoms of depression and anxiety. In the next chapter, I'll help you figure out whether symptoms of a possible mood disturbance are related to sleep deprivation, depression, or anxiety. But for the moment, it's important to be aware that disturbed or insufficient sleep can greatly affect your mood and overall mental health.

How Sleep Deprivation Affects the Brain

Besides experiencing changes in mood, some people with chronic sleep deprivation also notice that they have memory problems. Numerous studies have shown that sleep is crucial for intellectual functioning. For example, research has shown that sleep deprivation can cause significant deterioration in cognitive skills, such as attention and concentration, and motor functioning affected by mental processes, such as response time and eye-hand coordination (Kahol et al. 2008). In addition, academic performance in students is negatively impacted by sleep loss. This is because the ability to learn and retain information is affected by not getting enough sleep (Curcio, Ferrara, and De Gennaro 2006; Gibson et al. 2006). This means that studying or preparing for a work presentation or other important event shouldn't come at the expense of getting enough sleep. When you feel rested, you tend to think more clearly and have more energy.

Drowsy Driving: Are You at Risk?

Another important issue with regard to not getting enough sleep is driving. Media coverage of this issue has increased, and appropriately so, as the consequences of drowsy driving, or falling asleep at the wheel, can be fatal. If you've ever noticed yourself closing your eyes while at a stop sign or red light, then you're too sleepy to be driving. It only takes a few seconds of sleep (called a microsleep) to cause an accident. If you become sleepy while driving, pull over to a safe location and take a nap or call someone who can come and pick you up. Typical times of day when people become drowsy are in the middle to late afternoon and late at night. This is due to the natural biological rhythm that makes us sleepy at those times of day.

Drowsy driving is a problem not only because of the risk of falling asleep at the wheel, but also because you may have decreased reaction time and problems with attention. In fact, performance testing has confirmed that people who have chronic sleep problems, such as insomnia, have a slowed reaction time and impaired attention (Edinger et al. 2008).

Lack of Sleep Can Affect Your Weight

What about weight gain? Can insufficient sleep make it difficult for you to lose weight or even cause you to gain weight? Research over the past few years indicates this can occur and has identified two hormones involved in the process: leptin and ghrelin (Crispim et al. 2007; Copinschi 2005; Gangwisch et al. 2005). Leptin regulates your appetite by sending a signal to your brain to let you know when you've eaten enough and your stomach is full. When you don't get enough sleep, your leptin levels may decrease, making it more likely that you'll overeat.

Ghrelin, on the other hand, stimulates your appetite. Ghrelin levels may increase when you don't sleep enough, making you feel hungry more often. Of course, there are many other factors that contribute to weight gain, including diet, the amount of exercise and other activities you do, and certain medical conditions. However, it does appear that chronic sleep deprivation may play a role in making it difficult for people to lose weight or to maintain an ideal body weight. Since obesity is a risk factor for many different medical conditions, including obstructive sleep apnea, it's important for you to consider whether not sleeping enough could be affecting your weight, and therefore your overall physical health.

Medical Conditions Associated with Poor Sleep

Other physical problems that can be related to chronic sleep loss are hypertension (high blood pressure), cardiovascular disease, diabetes, and stroke. For example, shortened sleep time may impair glucose metabolism and increase the risk of diabetes, independent of its effect on weight or body mass index. Another way that chronic sleep loss may increase the risk of diabetes is through weight gain, which can cause insulin resistance (Knutson et al. 2007). Studies have also shown that chronic shortened sleep time may increase the risk of hypertension (Cappuccio et al. 2007; Gangwisch et al. 2006). Similarly, recent studies suggest that sleep disturbance may elevate risk for cardiovascular disease and stroke (Irwin et al. 2008), particularly for people with obstructive sleep apnea (Grigg-Damberger 2006).

In addition to increased risk for certain medical conditions, the less you sleep, the more likely you are to engage in behaviors that may be detrimental to your health in the long run, such as drinking excessive amounts of alcohol, smoking cigarettes, getting insufficient exercise, and making poor food choices. This is because when you're chronically short on sleep, you probably won't handle stress as well, so your coping skills decrease. In other words, when you feel stressed, sleep deprivation may lead you to grab a beer, eat some junk food, or smoke a cigarette, rather than taking a walk or relaxing in a hot bath.

Finding Out How Sleepy You Are

Some people with insomnia feel quite sleepy during the day, while others just feel drained of energy and fatigued. To find out how sleepy you are during the day, fill out the following questionnaire, entitled the Epworth Sleepiness Scale. It will help you assess how sleepy you typically feel when engaged in a variety of common daily activities. This questionnaire, which is frequently used in sleep centers all over the world, was created by Murray W. Johns in 1991 at Epworth Hospital in Melbourne, Australia (Johns 1991).

Epworth Sleepiness Scale

Name: _____ Today's date: _____

Your age (years): _____ Your sex (male = m; female = f): _____

How likely are you to doze off or fall asleep in the following situations, in contrast to feeling just tired? This refers to your usual way of life in recent times. Even if you haven't done some of these things recently, try to work out how they would have affected you. Use the following scale to choose the most appropriate number for each situation:

0 = would never doze

1 = slight chance of dozing

2 = moderate chance of dozing

3 = high chance of dozing

It is important that you answer each question as best you can.

Situation	Chance of Dozing
Sitting and reading	
Watching TV	
Sitting inactive in a public place (for example, a theater or a meeting)	
As a passenger in a car for an hour without a break	
Lying down to rest in the afternoon when circumstances permit	
Sitting and talking to someone	
Sitting quietly after a lunch without alcohol	
In a car, while stopped for a few minutes in traffic	

Scoring the Epworth Sleepiness Scale

A score between 1 and 6 indicates that you aren't sleepy during the day. A score of 7 or 8 is within the average range. A score of 9 or higher indicates that you are quite sleepy during the day and need to figure out why. A score of 18 or more means that you're very sleepy and need to take necessary precautions when feeling sleepy, such as not driving or operating machinery.

Are You Tired, Fatigued, or Sleep Deprived?

As you may have figured out by assessing yourself with the Epworth Sleepiness Scale, there's a difference between feeling sleepy and feeling fatigued. A lot of people with insomnia describe themselves as feeling fatigued during the day, but they still can't fall asleep if they try to take a nap. Fatigue is a feeling of being worn out or drained, either physically or mentally, whereas feeling sleepy indicates having trouble staying awake and alert. Of course, you may feel both sleepy and fatigued at any given time. Most insomniacs are fatigued, not sleepy, during the day. In the next chapter, we'll take a look at some other sleep disorders that may be causing you to feel sleepy.

Chronic sleep deprivation can decrease your performance at work and in other activities and make you feel sluggish or easily distracted. It can even affect your physical health, since many diseases are worsened by lack of sleep. So, why am I reminding you of the potential problems that can occur due to poor sleep? For motivation, because you need to take action now and do something about your sleep problem.

Perhaps you're wondering, "How many hours of sleep do I need anyway?" There's no clear-cut answer to this question. Different people need different amounts of sleep, so you shouldn't compare yourself to your friends, neighbors, family, or significant other. Instead, focus on how you feel during the day. If your energy level is good throughout the day without having to consume excessive caffeine, you're probably getting enough sleep at night. On the other hand, if you feel fatigued often or even just occasionally, you may be sleep deprived.

Assessing the Impacts of Your Sleep Problem

This exercise will help you examine how your sleep problem and the resulting sleep deprivation may be affecting the rest of your life.

___ yes	___ no	Do you ever stay home from work due to your poor sleep?
___ yes	___ no	Do you avoid social situations due to your poor sleep?
___ yes	___ no	Does your job performance suffer due to your poor sleep?

___ yes	___ no	Have you spent time and money on traditional treatments for your sleep problem, such as medications or doctor visits?
___ yes	___ no	Have you spent time and money on nontraditional treatments, such as acupuncture, herbal supplements, and aromatherapy?
___ yes	___ no	Have you ever fallen asleep or felt very drowsy while driving after a poor night of sleep?
___ yes	___ no	Is your attention and concentration worse after a bad night of sleep?
___ yes	___ no	Do you think your sleep problem has affected your relationships with family, friends, or significant others?
___ yes	___ no	Do you feel too tired during the day to exercise?
___ yes	___ no	Do you often feel tired or sluggish during the day?
___ yes	___ no	Have you gained weight recently or are you eating more than usual?
___ yes	___ no	Do you worry excessively about your sleep?
___ yes	___ no	Is your mood irritable or sad after a bad night's sleep?

If you answered yes to 1 or 2 questions, your sleep problem is affecting the rest of your life and it's important to start addressing your sleep issues. If you answered yes to 3 or 4 questions, your insomnia is already taking a moderate toll on your life. If you answered yes to 5 or more questions, your poor sleep is significantly impacting your life and it's very important that you focus on resolving your sleep problem. Fortunately, by continuing with the reading, exercises, and self-help techniques in this workbook, you'll be well on your way to sleeping better.

Short Sleepers and Long Sleepers

Some people, called *short sleepers*, need significantly less sleep than most of us to feel rested and well during the day. Others, called *long sleepers*, need much more sleep on a nightly basis to feel rested. According to the *International Classification of Sleep Disorders*, short sleepers routinely sleep five hours or less per day, without any noticeable decrease in daytime functioning (American Academy of Sleep Medicine [AASM] 2005). For short sleepers, decreased need for sleep is a natural occurrence; it isn't due to actively restricting or avoiding sleep, or to taking stimulants.

Long sleepers typically need ten hours of sleep or more per night to feel refreshed during the day. If long sleepers don't sleep as many hours as they need, they typically feel sleepy during the day. This longer sleep pattern usually begins during childhood, but social, occupational, and environmental factors may make it difficult for them to get as much sleep as they need. When this happens, they will experience daytime sleepiness or decreased daytime functioning, even if they get eight hours of sleep at night.

The amount of sleep you need can vary slightly from night to night. For example, if you're sick, you may need more sleep during this time due to feeling run-down and fatigued, and because of your body's need to rest and regain its strength. Similarly, if you've been exercising regularly, you may find that your body needs more sleep each night in order to feel rested. On the other hand, there may be occasions where you need less sleep, perhaps due to excitement about upcoming events, and you feel energized and well during the day. In chapter 4, I'll help you figure out how much sleep is right for you. The sleep restriction techniques in chapter 7 will also be helpful in this regard.

DISPELLING SLEEP MYTHS

Now that you've learned some of the basics about sleep, let's take a look at some common myths about sleep that may be contributing to your sleep problems.

Myth 1: Spending more time in bed at night will give me a better chance of falling asleep.
Actually, the opposite is true. The longer you spend in bed without sleeping, the more your mind and body will associate your wakeful state with your bed, thus making it harder for you to fall asleep. So instead of feeling more relaxed and sleepy when you get into bed each night, you're actually conditioning yourself to think of the bed as a place where you *don't* get good sleep. This simply leads to more frustration.

Myth 2: I need at least eight hours of sleep each night to be healthy.
This is not necessarily true, but it's easy to see why you may believe this. The media often misinterprets research data, or reports on only one finding of a study. Many different factors affect your health, and blaming lack of sleep as the sole culprit in poor health isn't medically sound. Although I do want to emphasize the importance of getting enough sleep, there's no "golden number" of hours of sleep that everyone must achieve each night in order to be healthy, both physically and mentally. As mentioned, the number of hours of sleep needed each night varies widely among people. The best indication of whether you're getting enough sleep is how you feel and perform during the day.

I remember one forty-three-year-old healthy woman who told me, "Ever since I was about twenty, I've slept around six hours per night and felt perfectly fine. I have plenty of energy during the day, and I'm doing very well at my demanding job. But now I'm always reading in the papers about how I should get at least eight hours of sleep at night. I don't want my health to be affected." In response, she started spending more time in bed at night, hoping that she'd get sleepy, but it just didn't happen. Luckily, she came to see me early enough that she avoided reinforcing a bad sleep habit that could have developed into a chronic sleep problem. Through education alone, she left my office feeling better and realizing that she didn't actually have a sleep problem.

Myth 3: A little nap during the day won't affect my sleep at night.
This is false. As mentioned before, everyone has individual sleep time requirements. Sleep is accumulated across a twenty-four-hour period, not just at night. So if you typically need seven hours of sleep at night to feel rested and well the next day, taking a one-hour nap during the day can reduce the amount you need that night to only six hours.

By the same token, if you're having trouble falling asleep or staying asleep at night, it's important not to nap during the day, as you'll only worsen your problems at night. Falling asleep is dependent on how sleepy you are and how many hours you've been awake prior to bedtime. If you nap during the day, it can affect both of these factors. The ability to fall asleep is also affected by social cues and your *circadian rhythm* (a roughly twenty-four-hour cycle of physiological, biochemical, and behavioral processes that are internally generated, but can be influenced by external factors).

Myth 4: Insomnia only happens to people who are anxious or depressed.

This is not true. Although depression or anxiety can certainly cause insomnia, so can plenty of other things. I'll cover this topic in greater detail in later chapters, so for now, please just be aware that insomnia can be caused by medical problems, other sleep disorders, medication side effects, poor sleep hygiene, and psychiatric disorders other than depression and anxiety. It can also exist on its own, as the only complaint that a person has. Although in the past sleep specialists and doctors were trained to believe that insomnia was always a symptom of something else, new research seems to indicate that this may not always be the case (Edinger et al. 2008; Richardson 2007; Mai and Buysse 2008). In other words, at times insomnia can occur on its own, entirely unrelated to psychiatric or medical disorders.

Myth 5: A few drinks before bed help me sleep better at night.

This is false. Although you may initially feel drowsy after drinking alcohol and find that you fall asleep more easily, alcohol can actually disrupt your sleep architecture and cause your sleep to be less restorative. You may end up tossing and turning in the latter parts of the night, or you may have to make a few extra trips to the bathroom. The bottom line is that alcohol is not a good sleep aid and shouldn't be used in this way.

Myth 6: Watching TV in bed helps me to fall asleep at night.

This is not true. Actually, your mind becomes activated when you watch television, assuming that you're paying attention to what you're watching. You experience both audio and visual stimulation, neither of which is conducive to good sleep. Although you might not have had a problem with watching TV in bed in the past, you've chosen to read this book because you want to improve your sleep. So you should watch TV in another room, not while lying in bed.

Myth 7: If I don't get enough sleep during the week, I can always catch up on the weekends.

Do you remember thinking this when you were growing up, especially as a teenager or a college student? Unfortunately, this isn't entirely true. Although you can sleep longer hours on the weekends and feel better on those days, this doesn't prevent you from being sleep deprived during the week. If your daytime functioning is poor during the week because you aren't getting enough sleep, sleeping for longer periods on the weekends will only make you feel better the following days. There is no catching up on lost sleep. Once it's gone, it's gone forever. It's important to realize that you can't burn the midnight oil, doing extra work or staying out late, and then expect to regain your lost sleep at another time. It just doesn't work that way. But don't despair over that thought, because this book will help you work toward getting restful sleep the majority of the time (which may require significant lifestyle changes).

I remember seeing a patient in New York who was a musician. He was in his thirties and played in bars and clubs late at night, often not going to bed until 4 or 5 a.m. He would then sleep for a few hours before having to get up and take care of things during the day, like paying bills, running errands, and seeing friends. He tried to catch up on sleep on his days off, but it didn't work for him. He was always tired because he simply wasn't getting enough sleep. Since he wanted to keep working as a musician and the only jobs he could find were at night, we devised a sleep schedule that allowed him to get at least seven hours of sleep daily without changing his bedtime and rising time on his days off. He felt much better with his new schedule and was also able to keep doing what he loved.

The point is, you shouldn't restrict your sleep voluntarily with the idea that you can get it back some other time. Although everyone may occasionally have a night or two of insufficient sleep, it certainly shouldn't become a regular habit. As mentioned before, the medical consequences of chronic sleep deprivation can be dangerous.

SUMMING UP

This chapter provided you with some basic knowledge about sleep. Now you're ready to learn about insomnia and start examining the factors that contribute to making it a good night versus a bad night. With that knowledge in hand, you'll be better equipped to get the restful sleep you need.

CHAPTER 2

What Is Insomnia?

Right now you may be asking yourself, "Why am I so tired all the time, and yet when I lie down, I just can't sleep?" The likely answer is that you've conditioned yourself to sleep poorly (a phenomenon I'll discuss at length later in the book). At some point in the past, due to stress or some change in your life (starting a new job, a short-term illness, and so on), you had some sleepless nights. You may know other people who have had the same problem, and they may all tell you not to worry, that your sleep will get better soon.

But what if the situation isn't getting better, and in fact, it's actually getting worse? You probably aren't even stressed about your new job anymore, or whatever it was that originally kept you up at night. But you're still losing sleep. And what's worse, you've probably developed some bad sleep habits. You may be spending more and more time lying in bed at night but getting less and less sleep. You may try to get yourself to bed just a little bit earlier each night, hoping you'll get the sleep you so desperately need. But if it were working, you wouldn't be reading this book. It may be that your sleep has gotten so bad that on some nights you just lie awake for what feels like an eternity, tossing and turning, hoping that you'll at least get a couple of hours of sleep before the sun comes up.

INSOMNIA OVERVIEW

Before you get started on the project of improving your sleep, it's important that you understand insomnia, its various subtypes, and typical symptoms. Although there are different definitions of insomnia from various authors, let's start by going directly to the diagnostic classification put out by the American Academy of Sleep Medicine in the *International Classification of Sleep Disorders*. There, insomnia is defined as "repeated difficulty with sleep initiation, duration, consolidation, or quality that occurs despite adequate time and opportunity for sleep and results in some form of daytime impairment" (AASM 2005, 1). Most people with insomnia have difficulty either falling asleep, known as *sleep onset insomnia*, or staying asleep, known as *sleep maintenance insomnia*. If you have insomnia, you may also have trouble functioning during the day. For example, you might feel irritable or short-tempered or have an overall bad mood. Other impairments may include feeling sluggish, being fatigued or tired, and having decreased attention and concentration. And what's worse, even though you may feel tired during the day, you probably can't sleep well at night or take a nap when you feel like you really need it.

Transient, or Acute, Insomnia

Transient, or acute, insomnia is a short-term sleep problem. It's actually quite common and usually occurs during stressful times, such as losing a loved one, moving to a new city, changing jobs, or ending of a significant relationship. Even seemingly joyous occasions, such as planning a wedding, graduating from college, or sending your child off to their first day of school, can cause stress and lead to insomnia.

Transient insomnia can also result from short-term illnesses; disruptions in the normal sleep schedule due to jet lag or working rotating shifts; environmental factors, such as light, noise, or temperature changes; certain medications, particularly those used for colds, allergies, asthma, and high blood pressure; and temporary physical or emotional discomfort or pain. In most cases of transient insomnia, the symptoms go away within a few days or a couple of weeks and don't cause long-term distress. Even so, you may find acute insomnia disruptive enough that you'd like to develop some skills for dealing with it. Perhaps you're worried that the next time you have a bout of transient insomnia it will turn into a more chronic problem that will impair your functioning. This workbook isn't just for those with long-term, or chronic, insomnia. It can also help you sleep better if you have transient insomnia and will help prevent your short-term insomnia from becoming a chronic, long-term problem.

Conditioned, or Learned, Insomnia

Unlike transient insomnia, which is short-term in nature and typically due to an identifiable stressor, in conditioned insomnia the stressful situation that initially caused your sleep disturbance may now be long gone, but you still have difficulty falling asleep or staying asleep—or both. It's important to put a stop to this type of problem. The longer you wait, the worse your insomnia is likely to become. Insomnia is considered to be chronic when it occurs at least three nights per week for a month or longer. (Technically, this type of insomnia is referred to as psychophysiological insomnia. It's discussed at length a bit later in this chapter.)

If you have conditioned insomnia, you may spend a lot of time thinking about your sleep problems, which leads to greater arousal at bedtime. So even as you start to prepare yourself for going to sleep, you actually feel more alert and awake and may have difficulty shutting off your mind. This increased level of arousal at bedtime is actually a conditioned physiologic response that contributes to difficulties falling asleep. In other words, people with psychophysiological insomnia have actually learned to sleep poorly. This can lead to impaired functioning during the day. The key is to stop this pattern as soon as you realize it's happening or causing a disturbance in your life.

If you have chronic symptoms of insomnia, your social and work life can suffer, especially if you spend much of the day concerned about your lack of sleep. Some people begin to limit their social activities, thinking that a night out with friends will only worsen their insomnia. Others feel that their performance at work is impaired. These issues can greatly affect your overall quality of life. In addition, lack of sleep may cause physical symptoms, such as headaches, increased muscle pain, and even stomach problems. But don't worry! This workbook can help you with your insomnia, whether it's a short-term or long-term problem.

INSOMNIA SUBTYPES

The *International Classification of Sleep Disorders* (AASM 2005) categorizes insomnia into the following subtypes:

- Adjustment insomnia (acute insomnia)

- Psychophysiological insomnia

- Paradoxical insomnia

- Idiopathic insomnia

- Insomnia due to mental disorder

- Inadequate sleep hygiene

- Behavioral insomnia of childhood

- Insomnia due to a drug or substance

- Insomnia due to a medical condition

- Insomnia not due to a substance or known physiological condition, unspecified (non-organic insomnia, not otherwise specified)

- Physiological (organic) insomnia, unspecified

You probably didn't know that sleep specialists have so many different ways to classify problems with sleeping!

If you haven't sought medical attention for your sleep problem and think that you may have insomnia, it's important that you see a physician who can evaluate you for possible underlying causes of your insomnia and make an accurate diagnosis. This is important for ruling out other illnesses, medication side effects, and so on. However, you may find that your doctor recommends sleep medications. If this happens, just remember that you *can* improve your sleep without medications. There are good reasons for doing so, which we'll explore at length in chapter 3.

HOW COMMON IS INSOMNIA?

If you're reading this book, it's likely that either you or a loved one is experiencing sleep problems. Unfortunately, statistics indicate that insomnia is a common problem. The National Institutes of Health

(2005) estimates that while about 10 percent of Americans actually meet the criteria for a diagnosis of insomnia due to trouble sleeping at night *and* impaired daytime functioning, up to 30 percent of the U.S. population has disrupted sleep. This means that 30 to 90 million Americans have problems sleeping at night. (For the purposes of this book, the term "insomnia" will be used more generally, to refer to sleep problems with or without impaired daytime functioning.) The prevalence of insomnia is high in the United States and industrialized countries worldwide, with some studies indicating that about 35 percent of the general population has insomnia (Sateia et al. 2000). According to the National Sleep Foundation's 2002 *Sleep in America* poll, 58 percent of adults in the United States had trouble sleeping a few nights a week or more. The poll found that insomnia is the most common sleep disorder among older adults, affecting 48 percent. In addition, some studies have shown that between 12 and 25 percent of healthy older adults have chronic insomnia (Morin, Colecchi, et al. 1999), with other studies reporting estimates as high as 57 percent in the elderly general population (Foley et al. 1995). The numbers are even higher for people who have psychiatric or medical illnesses.

In the 2007 *Sleep in America* poll, the National Sleep Foundation focused its study on women. They found that approximately 67 percent of women reported having a sleep problem at least a few nights per week within the past month, with 46 percent indicating a sleep problem every night or almost every night. In addition, nearly half of the women said they spent a lot of time awake during the night at least a few nights per week in the past month and that they generally wake up feeling unrefreshed. About one-third of women polled said they woke up too early in the morning and couldn't fall back asleep. Pregnant women and women who had recently given birth were even more likely than women in general to experience sleep problems at least a few nights per week.

There are significant public health consequences to this epidemic of poor sleep. Estimates of the costs associated with insomnia range from $92.5 billion to $107.5 billion annually (Stoller 1994). These high costs stem from more frequent doctor visits, missing days of work, increased use of prescription medications and over-the-counter drugs, and various other sleep-related treatments. As mentioned above, insomnia can also have a negative impact on quality of life, social functioning, and job performance. Plus, it can take a toll on family members, friends, and caregivers. Studies indicate that the prevalence and consequences of insomnia are actually underestimated because health care professionals lack sufficient knowledge about sleep-related issues (Sateia et al. 2000).

PSYCHOPHYSIOLOGICAL INSOMNIA

The most common type of insomnia for which people seek treatment is *psychophysiological insomnia* (briefly discussed above as conditioned, or learned, insomnia). To meet the criteria for psychophysiological insomnia, the person must have difficulty falling asleep or staying asleep for at least one month, with the sleep problem not being better explained by another medical, mental, neurological, or sleep disorder, nor due to medications or substance use. If you have psychophysiological insomnia, there is a conditioned component to your sleep disturbance. Over time, you've developed a heightened arousal at bedtime or while lying in bed, so you may feel wide awake when you're trying to fall asleep! People with psychophysiological insomnia often describe themselves as being unable to turn off their brains at night.

Does this sound familiar to you? Do you lie in bed thinking about things you have to do the next day or problems you're experiencing, or just worrying about when you'll finally fall asleep that night? If so, it's likely that you have psychophysiological insomnia.

Definition of Psychophysiological Insomnia

To further define psychophysiological insomnia, let's take a look at the criteria put forth by the sleep medicine world and the psychiatric field. The *International Classification of Sleep Disorders* (AASM 2005) notes that to have psychophysiological insomnia, you must have one or more of the following symptoms:

- You focus too much on sleep and have heightened anxiety about sleep.

- You have trouble falling asleep in bed at your desired bedtime or during planned naps, but have no problem falling asleep during boring or monotonous activities when you aren't trying to sleep (like at the movies or during a boring lecture).

- You sleep better when you're away from home (like at a hotel or a friend's house) than you do at home.

- You experience racing or intrusive thoughts or have a perceived inability to stop thinking or shut down your mind at bedtime.

- You have difficulty relaxing or feeling calm enough to fall asleep at bedtime.

The definition for psychophysiological insomnia was written by a group of sleep medicine researchers and experts. There's also a classification of insomnia from the psychiatric world. The *Diagnostic and Statistical Manual of Mental Disorders*, published by the American Psychiatric Association (1994), divides insomnia into four categories:

- Primary insomnia

- Sleep disorder related to another mental disorder

- Sleep disorder due to a general medical condition

- Substance-induced sleep disorder

The first of these, *primary insomnia*, is the near equivalent of psychophysiological insomnia. It's summarized as "a complaint of difficulty initiating or maintaining sleep or of nonrestorative sleep that lasts for at least one month and causes clinically significant distress or impairment in social, occupational, or other important areas of functioning" (American Psychiatric Association 1994, 553). As with psychophysiological insomnia, the diagnosis of primary insomnia is used when the problem isn't exclusively caused by another sleep disorder, mental illness, or the effects of a particular substance. The other types of insomnia listed in the *Diagnostic and Statistical Manual of Mental Disorders* can be grouped together as *secondary insomnia*. They're caused by other problems, such as pain, certain medications, health issues (like depression, heartburn, asthma, cancer, or arthritis), or substances such as drugs and alcohol.

To summarize, the term "insomnia" refers to difficulty initiating sleep, maintaining sleep, or waking up too early in the morning. If you experience any or all of these problems, you probably feel frustrated by your difficulties with sleep.

SECONDARY INSOMNIA

For many years, insomnia was considered a symptom and not a diagnosis in and of itself. Although there is now some evidence that insomnia can occur completely on its own, let's take a look at this idea of insomnia as a symptom. What this means is that insomnia can be caused by many different factors, and in order to resolve it, you need to figure out the root cause of the problem. To that end, the following sections will discuss some of the most common causes of secondary insomnia—depression, anxiety, medical conditions, medications, and other sleep disorders—and help you determine whether any of these are implicated in your sleep problem.

Depression and Insomnia

In people of all ages, insomnia can be related to depression or anxiety. Studies have found that 14 to 20 percent of adults with insomnia also have symptoms of major depression (Benca 2000). When evaluated in sleep labs, most people with depression show different sleep architecture than nondepressed people. For example, they have increased REM activity and an overall higher percentage of their total sleep time is spent in REM sleep. In other words, depressed people have more rapid eye movements while sleeping, and more eye movements during REM sleep than nondepressed people. As a result, depressed people typically spend less time in restorative slow-wave, or delta, sleep. They also go into their first REM period more quickly than nondepressed people. It's interesting to note that many antidepressants actually suppress REM sleep. In fact, research has found that sleep deprivation can actually improve the symptoms of depression, but obviously this isn't an appropriate or viable long-term solution (Benca 2000).

SYMPTOMS OF SLEEP DEPRIVATION VS. SYMPTOMS OF DEPRESSION

Not sleeping well can lead to mood changes. You may have noticed yourself becoming more irritable or on edge with others. Perhaps you no longer feel like the easygoing, even-tempered person you used to be. Everything may seem to bother you when you haven't had a good night's sleep. This isn't unusual; feeling irritable or short-tempered is quite common for people who are sleep deprived. Other symptoms of poor sleep include decreased motivation, poor attention and concentration, lack of desire to do things you used to enjoy, and not taking pleasure in things you used to enjoy. This last symptom, called anhedonia, is usually associated with depression. In fact, all of the symptoms mentioned above can also be symptoms of depression. Other symptoms of depression include sadness, hopelessness, feelings of guilt, decreased sex drive, and increased crying. However, these symptoms typically aren't associated with insomnia, so if you experience any of them, it's important to discuss them with your doctor.

Depression Checklist

To evaluate whether you're depressed, read through the following list and check off any symptom you experience, based on how you've felt during the past two weeks:

_____ You feel sad or down in the dumps most days.

_____ You find yourself crying more often than usual.

_____ There's been a change in your appetite.

_____ You have decreased energy.

_____ You're more irritable than usual.

_____ You have decreased attention and concentration.

_____ You feel sad or unhappy much of the time.

_____ You feel less motivated to do things.

_____ You enjoy activities less than you used to.

_____ You feel guilty more than you used to.

_____ You feel that the future is hopeless.

_____ You dislike yourself more than usual.

_____ You've lost interest in activities or other people.

_____ You're more fatigued than usual.

_____ It's harder to make decisions than usual.

_____ You have thoughts of killing yourself.

If you checked off at least five items, you have significant symptoms of depression. If you answered yes to having thoughts of suicide, it's important that you seek professional help immediately.

WHICH CAME FIRST, DEPRESSION OR INSOMNIA?

Many people wonder, "Is my depression causing me to lose sleep, or did my poor sleep cause my depression?" This can be a hard question to answer, and it often leaves even the best of sleep specialists puzzled and wondering what to treat first. So let's try to work it out together.

First, go back to the checklist in the previous exercise. Next to each symptom that you checked off, write down your best estimate of the date when that symptom began. You may not know the exact date, but try to remember as best you can. Once you've listed the dates next to your symptoms of depression, look at the checklist again. Did most of the symptoms begin around the same time? If so, when did you first begin to experience most of the symptoms? List the date or dates below (for example, "between Feb 15 and 25" or "around April 15"): _____

Now think of when you first started having trouble sleeping. When was this? List the approximate date below: _____

What came first, your symptoms of depression or your insomnia? _____

Were you able to find an answer to the question of which came first, your depression or your insomnia? If the majority of your symptoms of depression began before you started having insomnia, then depression may be causing your sleep problems. Have you had episodes of depression in the past? If so, did they always involve poor sleep? At times, insomnia can be the first sign that a person is depressed or the reason a person decides to seek help. If you haven't sought help for your depression, I highly recommend that you do so. With all of the various types of help available for depression, you don't have to endure these symptoms.

Although poor sleep may be due to depression, people with depression may also experience insomnia as a separate, unrelated problem. If you remember having sleep problems for a period of time before any other symptoms of depression appeared, then your insomnia may not be due to depression. Fortunately, the approach in this workbook can help you either way. You can benefit from treating your insomnia separately, even if you're suffering from depression or anxiety. Still, it's important to try to figure out whether your depression is causing your insomnia or your insomnia is causing your depression, so don't ignore symptoms of depression or anxiety.

According to the *Diagnostic and Statistical Manual of Mental Disorders* (American Psychiatric Association 1994), at least five depressive symptoms are required for a diagnosis of major depressive disorder. In addition, at least one of the symptoms must be depressed mood or loss of interest or pleasure in formerly enjoyable activities. If you've established that you do indeed have symptoms of depression, it's still important to try to differentiate cause from effect; that is, whether your depression caused you to have insomnia or your insomnia caused your depression.

Understanding How Your Insomnia and Depression Are Related

If depression is an issue for you, let's try to figure out whether you have primary, or psychophysiological, insomnia, in which your poor sleep is learned or due to conditioning, or secondary insomnia caused by your depression.

1. Which did you experience first, insomnia or depression? _____

_____

2.   How soon after your depression started did you experience insomnia (days, weeks, months), or how soon after your insomnia began did you notice symptoms of depression? _____

_____

3.   Does your insomnia seem to get better when your depression gets better? _____

_____

4.   Does your insomnia seem to get worse when your depression gets worse? _____

_____

5.   What other factors affect your insomnia? Consider the following examples: a stressful day at work; an argument with a friend, family member, or spouse; a short-term illness like the flu or a cold; worrying about finances; having a sick child; or going on a trip the following day. List those factors here, and consider whether any of them are always related to your depression.

_____

_____

_____

_____

_____

_____

Let's look at what your answers to each of these questions could mean.

For question 1, if you remember having symptoms of depression first, your insomnia is probably related to depression. However, if you remember having insomnia first, you can't immediately jump to the opposite conclusion—that insomnia caused your depression. As mentioned, sometimes insomnia is the first symptom of depression to appear. Many times, insomnia related to an episode of depression starts off as early morning awakenings. However, if the insomnia worsens and takes on a life of its own, it can lead to trouble falling asleep as well. The next question will shed more light on which came first.

Your answer to question 2 can provide helpful clues as to the source of your problem. If you noticed having insomnia first but started feeling depressed very soon afterward (within a few days or weeks), then it's likely that you had underlying depression that was first expressed through your sleep. This isn't unusual. If, however, a longer period of time passed between the onset of your insomnia and onset of other symptoms of depression, like a couple of months or more, then your insomnia may have caused you to develop symptoms of depression or they could be unrelated.

Similarly, if you started having insomnia soon after experiencing symptoms of depression, your insomnia is probably a result of depression. But if your insomnia developed months later, it could be an independent issue. If the insomnia seems to be independent of the depression, you need help that's specific to your sleep problem. Many people seek help specifically for their insomnia, even if they have had depressive symptoms off and on for years.

Questions 3 and 4 address this issue further, assessing whether the severity of your insomnia seems to be related to the severity of your depression. If you answered yes to either of these questions, it's likely that your depression is causing you to have insomnia. Ups and downs happen during the course of any major mental illness, including depression, and it's important to be aware of how this may be affecting your sleep. Having a better understanding of the ways depression impacts your sleep can increase your awareness so that you can take action to decrease the likelihood of this happening in the future. For example, you can make sure that you practice good sleep hygiene (see chapter 4) and utilize other helpful cognitive behavioral techniques you'll learn in this book. That way, your insomnia won't worsen to the point of taking on a life of its own, independent of your depression.

Lastly, let's take a look at your answer to question 5, about factors other than depression that affect your insomnia. This is important because many factors can affect your sleep. If you find that a number of them have nothing to do with depression, it's important to address those separate issues too. Environmental factors may be involved, such as loud noises, a baby crying, or a bed partner snoring. Or your insomnia may be exacerbated by other psychological factors, such as excessive worry and anxiety; medical problems such as pain, problems breathing at night, or gastrointestinal upset; or medication side effects. Try to think of all of the potential factors that may be contributing to your poor sleep, and go ahead and add them to the list above if you come up with additional items. Once you've done that, if your symptoms of depression still stand out as the greatest factor, then it sounds like that's what needs to be addressed first.

Anxiety and Insomnia

Insomnia is often related to anxiety, just like anxiety and depression may be related to each other. Anxiety is a normal emotion that we all feel at times, especially in stressful situations. In fact, feeling worried or nervous is a natural response to many types of difficult situations. But if you feel anxious most of the time, even in situations that don't appear to be stressful, then your anxiety is causing significant distress in your life. If so, it's important that you learn how to control your anxiety. Behavioral techniques such as deep breathing, relaxation exercises, and guided imagery can all be helpful. Cognitive restructuring can help you learn how to view situations differently and how to change your thoughts and reactions to various situations, which can also be useful in helping control anxiety.

Anxiety Checklist

Let's take a look at whether anxiety is an issue for you. Check off any of the symptoms listed below that you experience:

_____ Shortness of breath or difficulty breathing

_____ Racing heart or heart palpitations

_____ Excessive fear (of dying, of the worst happening, and so on)

_____ Difficulty relaxing

_____ Dizziness

_____ Feeling nervous much of the time

_____ Racing thoughts

_____ Uncontrollable, obsessive thoughts

_____ A choking sensation

_____ Nausea

_____ Difficulty staying calm

_____ Feelings of panic

_____ Ritualistic or compulsive behaviors (like hand washing)

_____ Feeling scared often or much of the time

_____ Frequent thoughts or flashbacks of traumatic events

_____ Frequent nightmares

_____ Trembling hands

_____ Frequent indigestion

_____ Hot or cold sweats

_____ Tingling or numbness in the feet or hands

_____ Feeling keyed up or on edge often

If you experience three or more of these symptoms often and they aren't always related to your sleep or a known medical condition, you may have an anxiety disorder. Do these symptoms cause significant distress in your life and affect your ability to function socially, at work, and in general? If so, it's important that you seek treatment for your anxiety in addition to working on your sleep problems. Cognitive behavioral therapy is very effective for anxiety disorders, and certain medications may be beneficial as well. Even if you do have an anxiety disorder, treating your insomnia is still very important.

Are You Anxious During the Day or Only at Night?

You've probably spent many hours worrying about your sleep. Is bedtime the only time of day when you feel anxious, or do you have anxiety at other times? Let's try to figure out how much anxiety affects your life.

2.   How often do you feel anxious?
     _____ Most of the day every day _____ Only at night _____ Occasionally during the day
     _____ A few times per week _____ Once a week or less

2.   What times of day do you feel anxious? _____ Only at night _____ Both night and day

3.   What kinds of things do you worry about during the day? (Check all that apply.)
     _____ Finances _____ Family _____ Health _____ Work _____ Relationships _____ Sleep
     _____ Other

4.   Is it difficult for you to relax? _____ Yes _____ No

Questions 1 and 2 ask how often and what times of day you typically feel anxious. If you answered "only at night" for either question, your anxiety appears to be focused primarily on your sleep. Many people believe that they only feel anxious at night, but once they start talking and thinking about it, they realize that they also feel nervous or anxious during the day. If you feel anxious most of the day, every day, you probably have an anxiety disorder that's separate from your insomnia. In this case, you should seek professional help specifically for your anxiety. If you experience anxiety occasionally during the day or less often, consider how much it's affecting your life. If it's impairing your quality of life, you owe it to yourself to get the help you need.

Question 3 asks about the focus of your anxiety. Is it only on sleep? Some people say that sleep is their only worry, but they still spend plenty of time worrying about it. It may be that your anxiety is focused solely on your sleep. However, if you often find yourself worrying about other things during the day, anxiety may be playing a bigger role in causing and maintaining your sleep problem. Even if you don't find yourself worrying much throughout the day, you may still lie in bed at night worrying about things you need to do the next day, work or family problems, or simply how many hours of sleep you're going to get that night. If you have psychophysiological insomnia, you're more likely to have intrusive and worrisome thoughts at night that prevent you from falling asleep.

Question 4 asks if you have difficulty relaxing. If you answered yes, is the problem only at night or does it occur during the day as well? If it's only hard for you to relax at night, particularly when you get into bed, then you've probably conditioned yourself to feel more alert and awake in bed, rather than the opposite. However, if you have trouble relaxing all of the time, it's likely that you're an anxious person with a sleep problem exacerbated by your underlying anxiety.

Whether or not anxiety is the cause of your poor sleep, it probably plays a significant role in maintaining it. Anxiety and insomnia are often related. Our goal is to end that relationship. By learning to think about sleep differently and engaging in sleep-promoting activities, you can improve the quality and quantity of your sleep.

Medical Diseases That Cause Insomnia

Many medical problems can affect sleep. If you suspect that you have any such medical conditions, it's important to see a qualified physician who can determine whether underlying physiological problems may be contributing to your disturbed sleep. Medical diseases that can cause insomnia include hyperthyroidism, dementia, certain types of cancer, and HIV. Allergies, asthma, and chronic congestion or coughing can also cause sleep problems. In addition, medications can exacerbate insomnia, even those taken for the common cold. People with chronic pain, arthritis, migraines, or fibromyalgia often have difficulty falling asleep, so adequate pain management is an important first step in those cases. If the pain is bad enough to wake you up during the night, it's especially important that you see a pain specialist for appropriate treatment.

Gastrointestinal illnesses are another source of concern. Acid reflux, also known as gastroesophageal reflux disease (GERD), can make it difficult to lie flat at night. Some people benefit from medication for this disease, while others are able to find relief by changing their diet or sleeping position. If you have acid reflux, limiting your consumption of caffeine and spicy foods can decrease discomfort at night that may make it difficult for you to rest. You may also find it helpful to avoid eating large meals at night and to avoid lying down after eating. Other gastrointestinal illnesses that can cause insomnia include irritable bowel syndrome and peptic ulcers. Irritable bowel syndrome can cause significant abdominal pain, which can make it difficult to fall asleep. This condition may also lead to more nighttime trips to the bathroom. Nocturia (urination at night) may cause frequent awakenings. In men, nocturia is often related to benign prostatic hypertrophy, while in women it's frequently related to stress incontinence, caused by weakness of the muscles of the pelvic floor. Stress incontinence may be improved by doing Kegel exercises or by taking medication. If those approaches fail, surgery may be an option.

Assessing the Role of Medical Conditions in Your Insomnia

Read through the following list of medical illnesses or symptoms that can cause difficulty falling asleep or staying asleep and check off any that you may have:

_____ Acid reflux

_____ Allergies

_____ Arthritis

_____ Asthma

_____ Cancer

_____ Chronic congestion or coughing

_____ Chronic fatigue syndrome

_____ Chronic or severe pain

_____ Dementia

_____ Fibromyalgia

_____ Frequent headaches

_____ Heart disease

_____ HIV

_____ Hypertension

_____ Hyperthyroidism

_____ Irritable bowel syndrome

_____ Migraines or chronic headaches

_____ Prostate problems

_____ Shortness of breath

_____ Ulcers

_____ Urinary frequency

If you checked off any of the symptoms or diseases on this list, it's important to ask your physician if this could be the cause of your insomnia. In many cases, treatment of the underlying disease or symptom is all that's needed to help people sleep well again. In addition, treating medical illnesses early can help avoid or minimize long-term complications.

Medications That Cause Insomnia

Many medications, both prescription and over-the-counter, can cause sleep problems. Herbal supplements may also interact with your sleep. Because some herbs are complex substances containing many compounds, and also subjected to less research than drugs, we don't know as much about how they affect the body. In addition, they aren't regulated by the Food and Drug Administration (FDA), so their quality and even their ingredients aren't assured. (I'll discuss some of the supplements most commonly used for sleep in chapter 3, on medications for insomnia.)

Assessing the Role of Medications in Your Insomnia

This exercise will help you assess whether medications play a role in your sleep problem. It lists common medications that can cause sleep disturbance. It isn't an all-inclusive list, but it does include the drugs most commonly prescribed for various health issues. For some medications, we have objective evidence about their effects on sleep because they've been researched in sleep labs. Other medications are listed because of subjective reports from patients who feel that insomnia is a side effect of that drug. It's important to keep in mind that while insomnia is a possible side effect of these medications, many people take them without experiencing sleep problems. However, it's important that you start taking a closer look at *all* of the things that could be disrupting your sleep, including any medications you take.

The following medications are listed by brand name, with the generic names in parentheses, where appropriate. Check off any medications that you take regularly:

Antidepressants

_____ Prozac (fluoxetine)

_____ Paxil (paroxetine)

_____ Zoloft (sertraline)

_____ Luvox (fluvoxamine)

_____ Celexa (citalopram)

_____ Effexor (venlafaxine)

_____ Wellbutrin or Zyban (bupropion)

_____ Lexapro (escitalopram)

_____ Cymbalta (duloxetine)

High blood pressure medications

_____ Inderal (propranolol)

_____ Toprol-XL (metoprolol)

_____ Lopressor (metoprolol)

_____ Tenormin (atenolol)

_____ Aldomet (methyldopa)

_____ Harmonyl (reserpine)

_____ Coreg (carvedilol)

_____ Normodyne or Trandate (labetalol)

_____ Cozaar (losartan)

_____ Apresoline (hydralazine)

Cholesterol medications

_____ Zocor (simvastatin)

Mevacor (lovastatin)

Questran (cholestyramine)

Colestid (colestipol)

Antiarrhythmic drugs

_____ Mexitil (mexiletine)

Tambocor (flecainide)

Cordarone (amiodarone)

Cardizem (diltiazem)

Corticosteroids

_____ Sterapred (prednisone)

Cortisol

Decadron (dexamethasone)

Bronchodilators

_____ Theo-Dur (theophylline or dimethylxanthine)

Ventolin or Proventil (albuterol)

Primatene Mist (epinephrine)

Parkinson's drugs (some are also used to treat restless legs syndrome)

_____ Sinemet (carbidopa-levodopa)

_____ Levodopa or L-dopa

_____ Eldepryl (selegiline or L-deprenyl)

_____ Symmetrel (amantadine)

_____ Mirapex (pramipexole)

Antiepileptic drugs

_____ Felbatol (felbamate)

Lamictal (lamotrigine)

Decongestants

_____ Pseudoephedrine

_____ Phenylpropanolamine

_____ Phenylephrine

Stimulants

_____ Desoxyn (methamphetamine)

_____ Ritalin (methylphenidate)

_____ Dexedrine or Dextrostat (dextroamphetamine)

_____ Provigil (modafinil)

_____ Cylert (pemoline)

Asthma medications (see Bronchodilators and Corticosteroids, above)

Thyroid medication

_____ Synthroid, Levothroid, Levoxyl, or Unithroid (levothyroxine)

Other Sleep Disorders That Can Cause Insomnia

Certain sleep disorders can also cause insomnia, including restless legs syndrome, periodic limb movement disorder, painful nocturnal leg cramps, circadian rhythm disorders, jet lag, shift work disorder, narcolepsy, obstructive sleep apnea, central sleep apnea, poor sleep hygiene, and environmental sleep disorder. Although parasomnias such as sleepwalking, sleep terrors, confusional arousals, sleep-related eating disorder, REM sleep behavior disorder, and nightmare disorder don't typically cause insomnia, they can be quite disruptive at night and possibly impact daytime functioning. Let's take a look at the characteristics of each of these sleep disorders so that you can determine whether any of them may be affecting your sleep.

RESTLESS LEGS SYNDROME

Restless legs syndrome (RLS) involves a painless creepy-crawly sensation in the legs that occurs in the evening hours, often at bedtime. It feels like an uncomfortable tingling sensation. Typically, the discomfort is relieved when the person massages their legs or moves around, but then the uncomfortable sensation slowly returns until they need to move their legs again. Typically, a person moves their legs in twenty- to sixty-second intervals at night, which can cause sleep onset insomnia. Caffeine and nicotine can make RLS symptoms worse, as can several types of antidepressants: selective serotonin reuptake inhibitors (SSRIs), monoamine oxidase inhibitors (MAOIs), and tricyclic antidepressants (TCAs).

If you have a creepy-crawly sensation in your legs at night and the uncomfortable sensation stops if you get up and move around or rub your legs, you could have RLS. There are both pharmacological and nonpharmacological treatments for RLS. The nonpharmacological approach includes taking a hot bath approximately one hour before bedtime, moderate daily exercise emphasizing the legs, and not using nicotine or caffeine. If you try this approach and it doesn't help your symptoms, seek the advice of a physician who's knowledgeable about RLS.

PERIODIC LIMB MOVEMENT DISORDER

Periodic limb movement disorder refers to an abnormal amount of limb movements during sleep. These may or may not be associated with brief awakenings that are typically not remembered. Many people affected by this disorder are unaware of having limb movements during sleep, but they may experience excessive daytime sleepiness and fatigue due to frequent arousals at night. At times, periodic limb movement disorder may make it difficult to stay asleep. As with RLS, symptoms can be worsened by caffeine, nicotine, and certain antidepressants. Pharmacological treatment is available.

PAINFUL NOCTURNAL LEG CRAMPS

Nocturnal leg cramps are sudden tightening, or spasms in the legs at night, usually in the calf muscles, but also in the feet or thighs. The cramps are painful and last from a few seconds to several minutes. They generally occur upon falling asleep or waking up, so they can cause sleep onset insomnia. If they occur during sleep, the pain can wake you up and cause sleep maintenance insomnia. Too much exercise or overuse of the muscles can cause these cramps, as can dehydration. Many pregnant women experience painful nighttime leg cramps, which may be due to calcium or magnesium deficiency. To prevent nighttime leg cramps from occurring, be sure to drink enough water during the day, and try stretching your legs, especially your calves, just before you go to bed. In addition, you may find it helpful to add more potassium, calcium, and magnesium to your diet. When a leg cramp occurs during the night, stretching or massaging your legs may relieve the pain.

ADVANCED SLEEP PHASE SYNDROME

Advanced sleep phase syndrome, sometimes called early bird sleep disorder, is a circadian rhythm disorder in which people are unable to stay awake until their desired bedtime or are unable to remain asleep until their desired wake time. In other words, people with this disorder fall asleep earlier in the evening than they would like to and wake up earlier in the morning than they want and are unable to fall back asleep. For example, someone who falls asleep at 8 p.m. each evening and wakes up at 4 a.m. may have advanced sleep phase syndrome. This syndrome is more common in the elderly but can occur at any age. Since it can be frustrating to wake up earlier than most people, people with advanced sleep phase syndrome may lie in bed trying to fall back asleep. This can lead to sleep maintenance insomnia.

DELAYED SLEEP PHASE SYNDROME

Delayed sleep phase syndrome, sometimes called night owl syndrome, is a circadian rhythm disorder with a pattern opposite that of advanced sleep phase syndrome: The person is generally unable to fall asleep until very late and has difficulty waking up at the desired time in the morning. For people with delayed sleep phase syndrome, the typical complaint is sleep onset insomnia, with extreme difficulty waking up in the morning at the desired time. Most often these people don't have trouble staying asleep once they've fallen asleep. This syndrome is more common in adolescents and college students but, like advanced sleep phase syndrome, may occur at any age. School performance may be impacted if a student experiences daytime sleepiness when attending morning lectures or while taking tests.

JET LAG

Jet lag is a disruption of the circadian rhythm in which sleep is disturbed and daytime alertness is impaired due to travel between time zones. Basically, it boils down to a mismatch between the sleep-wake cycle of your circadian clock and the sleep-wake pattern of the time zone to which you've traveled. This condition is only temporary, as the body can adjust its circadian rhythm to the new time zone within a few days. You may feel frustrated by a few sleepless nights after a long trip, but the problem usually resolves itself within one or two days. For people who travel often, like flight crews or frequent business travelers, poor sleep hygiene, negative or anxious thoughts about sleep, and increased frustration about sleep can cause temporary jet lag to develop into chronic, psychophysiological insomnia.

How bad the problem is and how long it lasts typically depend on the number of time zones you've crossed and the direction of travel. Traveling eastward, which requires you to advance your circadian rhythm and sleep-wake hours, is typically harder to adjust to than traveling westward. While some sleepiness after a long intercontinental trip may be caused by reduced sleep, it may also be caused by jet lag. As a rule of thumb, it takes one day to adjust for every two hours of time zones in an eastward direction, and one day to adjust for every three hours of time zones in a westward direction. For example, if you travel from New York to Geneva (eastward) in the springtime, there is a six-hour time difference, so it will take about three days to adjust to the new schedule. However, when traveling back from Geneva to New York (westward), it should only take two days to adjust.

SHIFT WORK DISORDER

Shift work disorder can occur when you work night shifts, rotating shifts, early morning shifts, or split shifts. This can result in insomnia when you try to sleep at atypical times of day, like during the daytime if you're a night shift worker. It can also cause excessive sleepiness during your work hours, since your body has a biological drive to sleep at that time. This disorder can lead to decreased productivity and performance at work, reduced alertness, increased accidents, and even personal problems due to the stress of having a different schedule from family and friends. People with shift work disorder find it difficult to sleep during the daytime hours, when most people are awake and active. Perhaps their sleeping environment isn't conducive to sleep because of noise, light, or household activity. In addition, people doing shift work may not be able to get enough sleep during the day because they have to take care of things like paying bills, going shopping, or picking up their kids from school. All of this can lead to sleep deprivation.

It's estimated that about 20 percent of the workforce in developed nations does shift work (Basner 2005). Although most of these people don't develop shift work disorder, for those who do, it's certainly a major problem. Behavioral treatment may be very effective for insomnia due to shift work disorder. For example, following some simple principles of good sleep hygiene, such as maintaining a regular bedtime and wake time, restricting caffeine and nicotine before bedtime, and keeping the sleeping environment quiet, dark, and comfortable can all make a big difference.

NARCOLEPSY

Narcolepsy is a rare sleep disorder that involves an unusually fast transition from wakefulness to REM sleep. This transition can occur during the day as well as at night. During the day, a sleep attack may happen suddenly, without any advance warning, and last only a short time. People with narcolepsy experience excessive daytime sleepiness and may also have cataplexy, a sudden loss of muscle tone caused by strong emotions such as fear, laughter, or surprise. Other possible symptoms include sleep paralysis (a feeling of being unable to move when falling asleep or waking up), hypnagogic hallucinations (very vivid perceptual experiences like seeing or hearing things that aren't there when falling asleep), and disrupted sleep at night. About 50 percent of people with narcolepsy complain of sleep problems, with sleep maintenance insomnia being more common.

Narcolepsy Questionnaire

Because suddenly falling asleep in the midst of daily activities can be problematic, if not hazardous, it's important to know if you suffer from narcolepsy. While this questionnaire won't definitively determine whether you have narcolepsy, it will indicate if it's a possibility.

___ yes	___ no	Do you have loss of muscle tone associated with heightened emotions, such as laughing, crying, or fear? (This isn't the same as fainting).
___ yes	___ no	Upon falling asleep or waking up, do you ever feel paralyzed?
___ yes	___ no	Do you ever see or hear things that aren't there (auditory or visual hallucinations) upon falling asleep or waking up?
___ yes	___ no	Do you frequently experience vivid dreams?
___ yes	___ no	Do you typically dream during short naps?
___ yes	___ no	Do you have sudden, uncontrollable urges to nap?
___ yes	___ no	Do you ever fall asleep without warning?
___ yes	___ no	Do you feel refreshed after napping for a short time, but feel sleepy again within two or three hours? And does this pattern repeat itself throughout the day?
___ yes	___ no	Do you have excessive daytime sleepiness?

These symptoms commonly occur in people with narcolepsy, but other people can experience them as well. The symptoms most indicative of narcolepsy include cataplexy, or loss of muscle tone associated with heightened emotions, and excessive daytime sleepiness. However, not everyone with narcolepsy will experience cataplexy. And while excessive daytime sleepiness is a hallmark symptom of narcolepsy, other sleep disorders can cause this symptom, including obstructive sleep apnea and periodic limb movement disorder. If you have any of the symptoms above and think you may have narcolepsy, you should discuss this with your physician so that you can obtain a definitive diagnosis. Narcolepsy and other sleep disorders causing these symptoms can be diagnosed by having your sleep evaluated in an accredited sleep laboratory.

OBSTRUCTIVE SLEEP APNEA

People with obstructive sleep apnea experience repeated episodes of complete obstruction of the upper airway (apnea) or partial obstruction (hypopnea) during sleep due to a collapse of the upper airway. (*Apnea* means cessation of breathing, and *hypopnea* is slow, shallow breathing that results in a reduction in airflow.) An episode of apnea or hypopnea typically lasts for at least ten seconds but can last significantly longer. These breathing problems typically cause the oxygen level in the blood to decrease. Snoring and excessive daytime sleepiness are the most common symptoms of obstructive sleep apnea, and some people with this condition awaken frequently and have difficulty staying asleep. Obstructive sleep apnea can cause serious consequences if left untreated and is also associated with other medical diseases.

The most commonly used treatment for obstructive sleep apnea is continuous positive airway pressure, a mask attached to a small portable machine that blows pressurized air into the airway to keep it open while the person is sleeping. Other treatments are available, but continuous positive airway pressure is considered to be the gold standard for treating obstructive sleep apnea. Some common causes of obstructive sleep apnea include being overweight or anatomical obstruction of the airway, such as enlarged tonsils, adenoids, or elongation of the uvula. Sleeping on your back can make obstructive sleep apnea worse for some people, so avoiding this position can be helpful for mild cases where the respiratory events tend to mainly occur while sleeping on your back. Weight loss is an important step in reducing your likelihood for obstructive sleep apnea. It's also a good idea for people with obstructive sleep apnea to avoid alcohol and sedatives prior to bedtime.

CENTRAL SLEEP APNEA

Central sleep apnea is a sleep disorder in which a person repeatedly stops breathing during sleep due to lack of respiratory effort. Whereas in obstructive sleep apnea the upper airway collapses, in central sleep apnea the brain doesn't send proper signals to the muscles that control breathing. There is a period of apnea that is sometimes followed by a period of hyperventilation, or rapid deep breathing. Central sleep apnea is much less common than obstructive sleep apnea and is usually associated with heart failure or conditions that affect the nervous system. It can also occur at very high elevations, typically above fifteen thousand feet. People with central sleep apnea typically complain of sleep maintenance insomnia, or difficulty staying asleep. The abrupt awakenings associated with central sleep apnea, which are often accompanied by shortness of breath can result in daytime sleepiness. Central sleep apnea requires medical attention and appropriate treatment. This may entail treating the underlying cause, using supplemental oxygen or positive airway pressure devices while sleeping, or taking medication.

Apnea Questionnaire

Both obstructive sleep apnea and central sleep apnea are serious medical conditions that can cause many complications. While this questionnaire won't definitively determine whether you have apnea, it will indicate if it's a possibility.

_____ yes	_____ no	Do you snore?
_____ yes	_____ no	If yes, is your snoring loud enough to wake others?
_____ yes	_____ no	Is your snoring worse when you sleep on your back?
_____ yes	_____ no	Do you ever awaken due to your own snoring?
_____ yes	_____ no	Has anyone noticed that you stop breathing during your sleep?
_____ yes	_____ no	Do you ever awaken gasping for breath?
_____ yes	_____ no	Do you have a choking sensation while sleeping?
_____ yes	_____ no	Do you cough frequently while sleeping?
_____ yes	_____ no	Do you feel very sleepy during the day?
_____ yes	_____ no	Do you have frequent awakenings at night?
_____ yes	_____ no	If yes, do you often need to use the bathroom then?

If you answered yes to any of these questions, particularly about stopping breathing during your sleep, you should discuss this with your physician so that you can obtain a definitive diagnosis. An overnight sleep test in an accredited sleep laboratory can determine whether apnea is an issue for you.

INADEQUATE SLEEP HYGIENE

Poor or inadequate sleep hygiene refers to unhelpful sleep habits that can interfere with falling asleep and staying asleep. Typical examples include consuming excessive amounts of caffeine, watching TV or reading in bed, using nicotine, exercising in the evening hours, and engaging in activities that are anxiety provoking or mentally stimulating prior to bedtime. If poor sleep hygiene is the problem, changing these habits will resolve the insomnia. It's unusual for poor sleep hygiene to be the main cause of chronic insomnia, but it's so easy to correct that it's worth addressing. Chapter 4 will give you the information and tools you need to improve your sleep hygiene.

ENVIRONMENTAL SLEEP DISORDER

Environmental sleep disorder is caused by disturbances in the sleeping environment. Common causes of this disorder include too much light in the bedroom; the temperature in the bedroom being either too hot or too cold; having a bed partner who snores, tosses and turns in bed, or kicks while sleeping; and noise from traffic, neighbors, barking dogs, or a crying baby. Environmental sleep disorder can cause either sleep onset insomnia or sleep maintenance insomnia. Once the environmental disturbance is eliminated, sleep should return to normal.

PARASOMNIAS

Parasomnias are behaviors that intrude into sleep, occur during transitions from one sleep stage to another, or occur during the transitions between sleep and waking (Rothenberg 2000). Generally considered to be undesirable at best, these behaviors either occur during sleep or are made worse by sleep (Kuhn 2001). Chapter 11 discusses some of the most common parasomnias. If the following exercise indicates that you may have a parasomnia, be sure to read the related section in chapter 11.

Parasomnia Questionnaire

This questionnaire will help you determine whether a parasomnia may be affecting your sleep problem. Alternatively, a sleep problem may make a parasomnia worse. In either case, it's worth identifying any parasomnias and taking steps to overcome them. Effective treatments are available for many of the parasomnias, and some may be resolved by relatively straightforward lifestyle changes. You'll find more information on parasomnias and treatments for them in chapter 11.

___ yes	___ no	1. Do you ever sleepwalk?
___ yes	___ no	2. Do you have frightening images during sleep that cause you to scream or get out of bed, but you typically don't remember these images in the morning? (These episodes aren't associated with dreaming.)
___ yes	___ no	3. Have you been told that you've done things during your sleep (other than sleepwalking) that you don't remember in the morning? Is your thinking confused or illogical at that time?
___ yes	___ no	4. Do you eat during your sleep but don't remember doing so?
___ yes	___ no	5. Do you ever act out your dreams?
___ yes	___ no	6. Do you have frequent nightmares?

If you answer yes to any of these questions, please be sure to read the section in chapter 11 relating to that particular symptom:

1. Sleepwalking

2. Sleep terrors

3. Confusional arousals

4. Sleep-related eating disorder

5. REM sleep behavior disorder

6. Nightmare disorder

Insomnia Questionnaire

The first step in overcoming your insomnia is to develop a better understanding of your particular sleep problem. This exercise will get you started:

1. Do you have trouble falling asleep after getting into bed? _____ yes _____ no

   If yes, how long does it usually take you to fall asleep each night? _____ minutes or hours

2. Do you wake up during the night after having fallen asleep? _____ yes _____ no

   If yes, how many times do you typically awaken each night? _____ times

   How long are your awakenings? _____ minutes or hours

3. Do you wake up too early in the morning? _____ yes _____ no

   If so, do you have trouble falling back asleep? _____ yes _____ no

4. What do you do during a typical awakening? (Check all that apply.)

   _____ Lie in bed _____ Use the bathroom _____ Watch TV _____ Watch the clock

   _____ Read a book _____ Worry about problems _____ Get up and walk around the house

5. Do you read or watch TV in bed? _____ yes _____ no

6. Do you talk on the phone or use your computer in bed? _____ yes _____ no

7. How many hours, on average, do you sleep each night? _____ hours

8. What is your usual bedtime?

   Weekdays: _____ a.m./p.m.

   Weekends: _____ a.m./p.m.

9. What time do you usually get up?

   Weekdays: _____ a.m./p.m.

   Weekends: _____ a.m./p.m.

10. Does your bedtime or rise time change by more than one hour from night to night or from week-nights to weekends? _____ yes _____ no

11. Are you bothered or worried by your sleep problems? _____ yes _____ no

12. Do you feel wide awake in bed? _____ yes _____ no

13. Do you experience racing thoughts in bed? _____ yes _____ no

14. Have you ever taken anything to help you sleep at night? _____ yes _____ no

    If yes, what have you taken? (Check all that apply.)

    _____ Over-the-counter medications such as Benadryl, Tylenol PM, Unisom, Equate, Sominex, Nytol, Sleep-Eze, Compoz, and Simply Sleep

    _____ Prescription sleep aids such as Ambien, Lunesta, Sonata, Halcion, Dalmane, Rozerem, Xanax, and Restoril

    _____ Dietary or herbal supplements such as melatonin, valerian root, chamomile, Calms Forté, passionflower, and hops

    _____ Alcohol or marijuana (for their sedating properties)

Questions 1, 2, and 3 are asking if you have trouble falling asleep or staying asleep, or if you wake up too early in the morning. If you answered yes to any of these three questions, you have symptoms of insomnia.

Questions 4, 5, 6 are asking about factors that may be making your sleep worse. These behaviors will be addressed further in upcoming chapters.

Questions 7, 8, 9, and 10 are asking about your total sleep time and your regular sleep schedule. If you aren't sleeping enough to feel rested during the day, your overall sleep time is probably too short. If your bedtime and rise time fluctuate from night to night and from weekdays to weekends, your sleep schedule may be contributing to your trouble sleeping.

Questions 11, 12, and 13 are asking about some typical symptoms of insomnia. If you answered yes to any of these questions, you will benefit from various skills and techniques in this workbook that will help you learn to sleep better.

Question 14 asks about your attempt to overcome insomnia by taking medications, either over-the-counter or prescribed, or by using herbal supplements, alcohol, or marijuana. Many people have tried medications or other substances to overcome their insomnia. However, there are significant drawbacks to this approach. This workbook offers an alternative approach—one that doesn't rely on medications or other substances.

SUMMING UP

Now that you have a good understanding of sleep and insomnia, and the possible reasons why you have trouble sleeping, let's move forward and start looking at solutions. Although medications are often the first recourse, they may not be the best solution. They often have unpleasant side effects, and they may not provide a long-term solution. In fact, the cognitive behavioral approach described in chapters 4 through 10 has proven to be a more effective long-term solution to sleep problems. However, because sleep medications are so widely prescribed and highly promoted, there's a good chance that you've already tried them, or that your doctor has encouraged you to try them. So before we get into the cognitive behavioral approach, let's take a look at sleep medications so that you can make an informed decision about whether to use them.

CHAPTER 3

Medications for Insomnia

The use of over-the-counter and prescription medications for sleep is very popular. It's estimated that between 5 and 12 percent of the general adult population uses medication to treat insomnia (Belleville and Morin 2008). The National Sleep Foundation (2007) found that 29 percent of women use some type of sleeping aid a few nights per week, and the numbers are also high in older adults, with sleeping pill usage estimated at 10 to 30 percent (Simon and Ludman 2006).

These numbers reflect the huge role that medications play in our society. Because pharmaceutical companies advertise directly to the public, you've probably seen many TV commercials telling you how wonderfully you'll sleep after popping a particular sleeping pill. But if you've tried to use medication to solve your sleep problem, you've probably wondered how long you'd need to keep taking the medication. Many people don't want to take sleeping pills for the rest of their lives, and this may be the case for you. Or perhaps you found that sleeping pills worked fine for you in the past, but they're no longer as effective. That's actually quite common, because your body can develop a tolerance to sleeping medications. Plus, the monetary expense involved in taking sleeping aids for a long time can be considerable. These are just a few of the many reasons why you may not want to take sleeping pills.

Most medications prescribed as sleep aids fall into the category of *sedative-hypnotic drugs*, which are central nervous system depressants. Since they are sedating in nature, they can be used as muscle relaxants, antianxiety medications, and to promote sleep. Although the majority of people who are prescribed these medications are having trouble sleeping as their main problem, sedative-hypnotics may also be prescribed for sleep problems associated with hypertension, depression, anxiety, heart disease, diabetes, congestive heart failure, airway obstruction, bronchitis, sinusitis, migraines, headaches, and psychotic disorders (McCall, Fleischer, and Feldman 2001). This is because many different medical conditions can interfere with sleep or cause increased anxiety and tension. In other words, you may be prescribed sedative-hypnotic medications for a whole bunch of different reasons, only one of which is a primary diagnosis of insomnia. If you're taking sedative-hypnotics and aren't sure why, ask your doctor why these drugs were prescribed for you.

In the rest of this chapter, you'll learn about the different types of prescription medications, over-the-counter drugs, and herbal remedies used for insomnia. I'll also explain the potential side effects of medications used for sleep, what you can expect if and when you decide to stop taking them, and techniques for discontinuing their use.

NONPRESCRIPTION OR OVER-THE-COUNTER SLEEPING AIDS

If you go to your local drugstore, health food store, or supermarket, you will surely find a variety of over-the-counter medications intended to help you sleep better. In general, the over-the-counter medications commonly used for sleep fall into two main categories: antihistamines (a class of drugs commonly used for symptoms of allergies, colds, or the flu) and supplements, including herbal remedies.

Antihistamines

Antihistamines are regulated by the Food and Drug Administration (FDA). Many of them are available over the counter, so it isn't necessary to have a doctor's prescription to purchase them, whether for sleep or for symptoms like a runny nose, itchy and watery eyes, and sneezing. Some antihistamines help prevent motion sickness or relieve itchiness caused by poison ivy, poison oak, or insect bites and stings. If you've ever taken an antihistamine, you probably experienced one of their most common side effects—drowsiness—explaining why they're so commonly used for insomnia.

Older antihistamines contain ingredients such as diphenhydramine (Benadryl, Sominex, Nytol, Tylenol PM, Advil PM, Excedrin PM, Compoz, Unisom, Equate, Sleep-Eze, Simply Sleep, and so on), doxylamine (Alka-Seltzer Plus Night Cold Medicine or NyQuil), dimenhydrinate (Dramamine Original), chlorpheniramine (Singlet), or brompheniramine (Lodrane 12 Hour, Dimetane, or Dimetapp Cold and Allergy). Some newer over-the-counter antihistamines contain loratadine (Claritin or Alavert) or cetirizine (Zyrtec). The older antihistamines are more likely to make you sleepy than the newer ones. The major active (and inactive) ingredients are listed on the packaging of all FDA-regulated medications sold in the United States, so you can see for yourself if a medication you take contains an antihistamine. Diphenhydramine is the antihistamine most commonly used for insomnia, but it definitely has drawbacks, including worsening the side effects of other drugs (McCall 2004).

Although antihistamines may help you fall asleep when you first start taking them, you may develop a tolerance to them, so they're no longer as effective at promoting sleep (Neubauer 2007). They may also make you feel groggy in the morning, since their sedative effects may last longer than you sleep. Other potential side effects include dry mouth, blurred vision, urinary retention, feeling dizzy and light-headed when standing up, confusion, constipation, palpitations, increased appetite, and cognitive impairment, such as memory problems and delirium (Neubauer 2007; McCall 2004). Due to insufficient evidence that antihistamines actually improve the symptoms of insomnia, they aren't recommended as a first-line treatment for sleep problems (National Institutes of Health 2005).

Supplements and Herbal Remedies for Sleep

Supplements commonly used for sleep include melatonin, valerian root, and kava. Other popular herbal remedies include passionflower, skullcap, lavender, chamomile, and hops. In the United States, herbs need not be tested for effectiveness or safety. And because they aren't regulated by the FDA, you can't be sure of the purity, concentration, or composition of herbs and herbal formulas, or how consistent the processing and manufacturing are. This means it's impossible to know if you're actually getting what you think you are when you buy an herbal product. For example, when valerian products were tested by a consumer agency, four out of seventeen products didn't even contain a detectable level of valerian. Another four products contained half of the amount indicated on the package, and one was contaminated with cadmium, a poisonous metal (Shimazaki and Martin 2007). This example isn't meant to scare you, but simply to illustrate the potential downsides of herbal products due to their not being regulated or tested to ensure their quality or safety. This lack of quality control means that product information and labeling can be misleading, and that certain herbal products can even be dangerous.

MELATONIN

Melatonin is a hormone that's naturally produced in the brain by the pineal gland. It's secreted at night, when it's dark. Since it helps to regulate the sleep-wake cycle of your circadian rhythm, supplemental melatonin can be helpful for occasional jet lag, shift work disorder, and delayed sleep phase syndrome, since the circadian rhythm is affected in all of these sleep disorders. It can also be helpful for blind people with sleep problems. However, supplemental melatonin has not been proven effective for insomnia per se (Neubauer 2007; National Institutes of Health 2005; Park et al. 2007). Despite the lack of evidence showing its usefulness for insomnia, it has become popular as a sleep aid. In the United States, about 5 percent of people use melatonin, with close to 28 percent of these people taking it specifically for insomnia (Bliwise and Ansari 2007).

The idea that melatonin is naturally produced by the body may lead you to think it's a good alternative to prescription sleep medications. However, supplemental melatonin may not be so benign. In fact, in some European countries melatonin is regulated as a prescription supplement and isn't sold over the counter (Guardiola-Lemaitre 1997) due to concerns about potential side effects. For example, there have been reports of melatonin causing vascular side effects, such as increased blood pressure and heart rate in people taking medications for high blood pressure (Lusardi, Piazza, and Fogari 2000), as well as changes in heart rate in healthy people (Vandewalle et al. 2007). Some researchers are also concerned about the possible effects of long-term use of melatonin on fertility, but that question remains unanswered (Weaver 1997). In addition, there is some evidence that supplemental melatonin can affect glucose tolerance and insulin sensitivity (Cagnacci et al. 2001), thus causing prediabetes. Since melatonin hasn't been proven to provide much relief for insomnia (other than circadian rhythm disorders), carefully weigh its risks and benefits if you're considering taking it.

VALERIAN

Another popular herbal remedy for insomnia is valerian root. Similar to melatonin, it isn't regulated by the FDA, so valerian products generally aren't standardized or tested for quality, purity, concentration, or composition. The active component in valerian is unknown, but it does appear to have a mild hypnotic effect while also helping reduce anxiety and relax the muscles. Despite these actions, there is a lack of convincing evidence that valerian helps with insomnia or has any true benefit in improving sleep (Neubauer 2007). It is estimated that close to 6 percent of the U.S. population uses valerian, with about 30 percent of these people taking it specifically as a sleep aid (Bliwise and Ansari 2007).

As with melatonin, it's important to consider the possible risks. Numerous studies have shown that herbs and other botanical supplements can interact with medications used for cardiovascular disease, diabetes, seizures, and cancer, as well as psychotropic medications (Bliwise and Ansari 2007). The effectiveness of valerian for insomnia is a subject of debate, but at the present time, there's insufficient evidence that it promotes sleep, so it isn't recommended as a treatment for insomnia (National Institutes of Health 2005).

KAVA

Sold as an herbal or dietary supplement in the United States, kava is a bitter herb derived from the fibers of a plant in the same family as black pepper. It's native to the western Pacific region, where indigenous cultures have used it for over three thousand years as a traditional recreational drink due to its relaxing properties. Kava is typically used for nervousness, anxiety, and stress, but its mechanism of action currently isn't known (Boon and Wong 2003). Once again, because it isn't regulated by the FDA, its concentration, potency, and quality vary greatly depending on the manufacturer.

There have been reports of some serious health problems due to kava use, including liver toxicity resulting in liver failure, cirrhosis, and hepatitis (Lude et al. 2008; Fu et al. 2008). Other potential adverse effects include dry, flaky, yellow skin, as well as hair loss, hearing loss, anorexia, muscle weakness, and problems with coordination (Wooltorton 2002a, 2002b). Due to significant drug interactions and effects on various mechanisms in the body, kava isn't recommended if you're taking antiplatelet medications, such as Plavix (clopidogrel) or aspirin; anticoagulant medications, such as Coumadin (warfarin); or antipsychotic medications; or if you have Parkinson's disease (Wooltorton 2002b). In 2002, both the FDA and Health Canada issued federal advisories warning people to stop taking kava until further information about its safety and possible liver toxicity were determined (Mills et al. 2004).

PRESCRIPTION SLEEPING AIDS

The medications used for insomnia have changed over the past fifty years. They have become significantly safer than in the days of barbiturates and chloral hydrate. Due to safety concerns and the potential for abuse with those older medications, pharmaceutical companies worked to develop and test alternatives that would be less harmful.

As mentioned, the number of people taking prescription sleep aids is quite high. With the allure of the numerous television ads for medications that promise more restful, peaceful sleep, it's easy to see why people might think that taking a sleeping pill could be the answer. Although these commercials try to convince people that they *need* a prescription sleep aid for insomnia, the reality is that the American Academy of Sleep Medicine recommends nonpharmacological approaches as the first step in overcoming a sleep problem. One reason is that you can become dependent on most sedative-hypnotics. *Psychological dependence* occurs when you think you can only fall asleep with the drug and therefore are scared or unwilling to stop taking it. *Physiological dependence* occurs when your body has adapted to the substance and actually needs that substance to feel normal. *Tolerance*, in which you need to take increasing amounts of the drug to obtain the same effect, is also cause for concern.

Because sedative-hypnotics can cause dependence, they aren't supposed to be taken long term, despite what some of the more recent commercials may advertise. And in truth, nonpharmacological interventions for insomnia, like those you'll learn in this book, are more effective in the long run. The first step in overcoming dependence on a sedative-hypnotic is to believe that you can learn to fall asleep on your own without the medication. Although this and the other techniques I'll describe require work on your part, it will be well worth it in the end when you no longer need to rely on a drug in order to fall asleep. These approaches will allow you to address the root causes of your sleep problem, overcome your insomnia, and not have it re-occur on a night when you don't take your sleeping pills, a problem known as *rebound insomnia*.

The current prescription medications available for the treatment of insomnia include benzodiazepines, nonbenzodiazepine hypnotics, ramelteon (Rozerem), barbiturates, antidepressants, and antipsychotics. Only some of these are approved by the FDA specifically for insomnia. Others have been approved for other conditions or diseases, but are quite commonly prescribed for insomnia, a practice known as *off-label use*. They too can be effective as sleep agents for some people. After the following discussion of the various categories of prescription sleep medications, you'll find a table summarizing key information about the most common sleep aids.

Benzodiazepines

Most sleeping medications come from the benzodiazepine class of drugs. In this class, only temazepam (Restoril), flurazepam (Dalmane), estazolam (ProSom), quazepam (Doral), and triazolam (Halcion) are approved by the FDA as a treatment for insomnia. Off-label use is quite common with benzodiazepines, however, so other drugs in this class are commonly prescribed for insomnia, including clonazepam (Klonopin), diazepam (Valium), alprazolam (Xanax), and lorazepam (Ativan). The main differences between the various benzodiazepine medications are the rate of absorption into the bloodstream, rate of distribution throughout the body, and how long the drug will stay there. If a drug is absorbed rapidly, its effects are felt rather quickly, which is more useful for sleep onset insomnia, or trouble falling asleep. If a drug has a slower absorption rate, it will take longer for the effects to be felt, so these types of benzodiazepines are more helpful for sleep maintenance insomnia, or trouble staying asleep.

Some drugs take longer than others to work their way out of your system, depending on their *half-life* (the amount of time it takes for your body to break down or eliminate half of the original concentration of the drug). This is important to know, because if a drug has a long half-life, it will continue to exert its effects longer than drugs with a shorter half-life. If a drug has a long half-life, you may still feel its effects the next day. This is commonly called a "hangover effect" because you may feel drowsy, groggy, or less clear-headed. Another factor that's involved in how long a drug affects you is the way it's metabolized or broken down in your body. Some drugs are metabolized quickly, but their breakdown products have effects similar to those of the drug you initially ingested, prolonging the duration of the drug's effects.

Benzodiazepines can impair your memory and performance, make you feel sedated in the daytime, and depress your mood (Spielman and Anderson 1999). In addition, they can decrease your respiratory functioning, so they aren't advised if you snore or have sleep-disordered breathing, such as sleep apnea. Benzodiazepines can affect sleep architecture by suppressing restorative stage N3 sleep and increasing spindle activity in stage N2 sleep (Mendelson 2000).

The biggest problems with benzodiazepines are that your body can become dependent on them or develop a tolerance to them. For these reasons, they're classified as schedule IV drugs by the U.S. Drug Enforcement Agency. Symptoms of withdrawal from benzodiazepines include rebound insomnia, agitation, anxiety, and, in more severe cases, seizures. These drugs have antianxiety, sedative-hypnotic, and anticonvulsant properties (Morin 1993), so when you stop taking them, your body experiences the opposite effect: increased anxiety, more trouble sleeping, and possibly even seizures. You should only stop taking benzodiazepines under careful medical supervision and guidance, as you're likely to need to decrease the dosage in a stepwise fashion, and even then you must be alert to possible symptoms of withdrawal.

Nonbenzodiazepine Hypnotics

Nonbenzodiazepines are a class of sedative-hypnotic drugs that first became available in the United States in the early 1990s. The first drug in this class was zolpidem (Ambien), with zaleplon (Sonata) and eszopiclone (Lunesta) following about a decade later. Their actions in the body are similar to those of the benzodiazepines, but they're more specific, being more selective with regard to which neurotransmitters they target in the brain. The benefit is that these newer drugs are more tolerable than the benzodiazepines, with decreased adverse side effects, decreased withdrawal effects when discontinued, and a lower potential for dependency (Neubauer 2007; Park et al. 2007). However, there is still some potential for dependence or abuse, so they're also classified as schedule IV drugs, like the benzodiazepines.

AMBIEN

Ambien (zolpidem), which is prescribed in either 5 or 10 mg dosages, is rapidly absorbed, so it starts working rather quickly. It has a half-life of 1.5 to 2.4 hours, meaning it will take that much time for the concentration of the drug in your body to be at half the level it was shortly after you took the drug. In other words, if you take 10 mg of Ambien at bedtime, after 1.5 to 2.4 hours, you'll have only 5 mg in your blood. After another 1.5 to 2.4 hours, the concentration decreases by half once again, to 2.5 mg. This makes it more effective at helping those who have trouble falling asleep. Given its half-life, its effects may last long enough to decrease awakenings during the night, but maybe not. To make the drug more helpful for those with sleep maintenance insomnia, a continuous-release form, Ambien CR, was developed. In this form, the drug is slowly released and absorbed in the intestinal tract over a longer period of time. Ambien CR is prescribed in doses of 6.25 mg or 12.5 mg. Unlike the benzodiazepines, Ambien doesn't appear to have significant effects on sleep architecture.

In the past few years, there has been considerable media attention on the possible adverse side effects of Ambien, including "sleep driving" and "sleep eating," in which people have no recollection of these events the following morning. The Ambien website and the drug's product information now list these unusual nighttime activities as possible side effects of taking the drug. Although the literature on Ambien discusses its lower potential for abuse compared to benzodiazepines, it's important to note that Ambien can be misused and abused. There are cases of people who take as much as 50 or 60 mg of Ambien per night because they say the drug is no longer working for them at the lower, prescribed dosages. This points to the importance of being cautious about using any sedative-hypnotic medication. Always seek professional help if you find yourself using more than the recommended dosage of your medication, or even wanting to use higher doses.

SONATA

Like Ambien, Sonata (zaleplon) is typically used for sleep onset insomnia. Available in dosages of 5 mg and 10 mg, Sonata has a rapid onset and absorption rate and is quickly eliminated from the body. The half-life is only about an hour. If you have sleep maintenance insomnia, Sonata won't be helpful because its effects will have already worn off. As with other sedative-hypnotics, taking Sonata on a nightly basis can lead to psychological or physiological dependence on the drug.

LUNESTA

Lunesta (eszopiclone), which is available in doses of 1 mg, 2 mg, and 3 mg, has a longer half-life than either Sonata or Ambien. Since it is rapidly absorbed and has a half-life of five to seven hours, it can be effective for both sleep onset insomnia and sleep maintenance insomnia. However, its longer half-life means it's more likely to cause daytime sleepiness or a hangover effect. Although the FDA has approved it for long-term use, it has the same risks of dependence as other sedative-hypnotics. Plus, since it is a relatively new drug, long-term use of Lunesta hasn't been extensively studied.

The most commonly reported side effects of Lunesta are headaches, an unpleasant taste in the mouth, infection, nausea, pain, unpleasant dreams, and sore throat. Side effects of Lunesta use include daytime sleepiness and depression (Brielmaier 2006; Lieberman 2007). Rebound insomnia can also occur, especially on the first night after discontinuing its use (Lieberman 2007). A similar drug, zopiclone (Imovane), is sold in Canada and Europe. It's an isomer of eszopiclone (Lunesta), meaning it has the same chemical formula but a different physical structure. Studies have shown that zopiclone can cause dependence, with withdrawal symptoms such as rebound insomnia, anxiety, heart palpitations, increased heart-rate, tremor, and seizures (Cimolai 2007).

Ramelteon

The newest sedative-hypnotic to be approved by the FDA for sleep onset insomnia is ramelteon (Rozerem). It targets two types of melatonin receptors in the brain that are thought to be involved in the regulation of the sleep-wake cycle of the circadian rhythm. One of the receptors is thought to regulate sleepiness, while the other is believed to help the body make the shift between daytime and nighttime (Kato et al. 2005; Zammit et al. 2007). Ramelteon is rapidly absorbed and has a half-life of 1 to 2.6 hours. It's highly selective and exerts much stronger effects than supplemental melatonin. In one large study, there was no evidence of rebound insomnia or other withdrawal effects after five weeks of use (Zammit et al. 2007). Possible side effects of ramelteon include headaches, daytime sleepiness, dizziness, and fatigue. Unlike the benzodiazepines and nonbenzodiazepines, ramelteon is classified as nonscheduled by the Drug Enforcement Agency, because it hasn't shown any potential for abuse. In fact, it's currently the only nonscheduled prescription sleep aid sold in the United States.

Barbiturates

Drugs in the barbiturate class of medications work as central nervous system depressants. In other words, they're sedating. In the past, barbiturates such as pentobarbital (Nembutal), secobarbital (Seconal), amobarbital (Amytal), and a secobarbital-amobarbital combination called Tuinal were used quite often as sleeping medications. The barbiturates prescribed for sleep are short-acting or intermediate-acting, meaning they begin working fifteen to forty minutes after being taken, and their effects can last from five to six hours. Even longer-acting barbiturates, such as phenobarbital (Luminal) and methylphenobarbital (Mebaral) have been used for insomnia; these cause sedation within one to two hours and their effects can last twelve hours or longer (Ray and Ksir 1993). There are several reasons why barbiturates are rarely used for insomnia anymore. First of all, barbiturates can be quite dangerous, as evidenced by the fact that some of them are classified as schedule II drugs, a category that also includes morphine, opium, and methamphetamine. Not only are they highly addictive, they also have more side effects, including a hangover effect, daytime sleepiness, and impaired muscle coordination for up to a day after taking a single dose. Tolerance, psychological dependence, and physical dependence are all common with these drugs. In addition, barbiturates depress respiration and can cause you to stop breathing. Taken in high doses or in combination with alcohol, they can be lethal (Schilit and Lisansky Gomberg 1991; Ray and Ksir 1993). To sum up, barbiturates are not recommended for insomnia.

Antidepressants

Some antidepressants have a sedating effect, explaining why they're frequently used in lower doses as sleep aids. People don't tend to develop tolerance to antidepressants to the same degree as they would to benzodiazepines or other hypnotics. Antidepressants often used for insomnia include doxepin (Sinequan), amitriptyline (Elavil), mirtazapine (Remeron), nefazodone (Serzone), and trazodone (Desyrel). Daytime sedation is sometimes a problem with these medications (Hauri 1998). Other possible side effects include dry mouth, trouble urinating, light-headedness, constipation, dizziness upon standing, heart rhythm irregularities, and impotence. In addition, certain antidepressants can exacerbate symptoms of restless legs syndrome or periodic limb movement disorder, so these sleep aids would be a particularly poor choice if either of these conditions affects your sleep.

The use of antidepressants for sleep is considered off-label, as they aren't approved by the FDA for insomnia. If you have depression in addition to insomnia, the more sedating antidepressants may be helpful for your symptoms. However, there is a lack of evidence showing that they improve sleep for those who don't suffer from depression, so their use in those cases is considered controversial (Holbrook 2004). Since there can be significant adverse side effects on antidepressants, you should carefully weigh the risks and benefits if you're considering using them for sleep (National Institutes of Health 2005; Neubauer 2007).

Antipsychotics

Antipsychotic medications are sometimes used for people who have insomnia along with another psychiatric disorder that would benefit from these drugs, such as mania, significant anxiety, or psychotic symptoms (Park et al. 2007). These drugs fall into two classes: typical and atypical. The typical antipsychotics used for their sedating properties are thioridazine (Mellaril) and chlorpromazine (Thorazine), and atypical antipsychotics used as sleep aids include quetiapine (Seroquel), olanzapine (Zyprexa), clozapine (Clozaril), and risperidone (Risperdal). Side effects associated with long-term use of typical neuroleptics include tardive dyskinesia, which is characterized by repetitive, involuntary, purposeless movements. Other side effects of typical antipsychotic medications include dry mouth, muscle cramping and stiffness, tremors, and weight gain. The newer atypical antipsychotics have been around for fewer years, so it's unclear if long-term use could cause tardive dyskinesia. Feelings of restlessness and an inability to sit still or remain motionless, along with anxious agitation, have been noted with both the older and newer antipsychotic medications. Weight gain is a common side effect of the atypical antipsychotic medications, as are low blood pressure and sexual dysfunction. In addition, there may be an increased risk of type 2 diabetes with the atypical antipsychotics, and there have been reports of an increased risk of stroke when used by the elderly (Gardner, Baldessarini, and Waraich 2005). Most people are prescribed antipsychotics for a psychiatric disorder, and they can be very effective for these problems; if that's the case for you, the benefits of these medications may very well outweigh their risks.

The following is a list of medications commonly prescribed for sleep. Since barbiturates and antipsychotics carry significant potential risks in comparison with other sleep aids, they are not recommended in the treatment of insomnia and are not included in this list.

Medications Commonly Used for Insomnia

Generic Name	Brand Name	Class	Dose (mg)	FDA-Approved for Insomnia?
alprazolam	Xanax	benzodiazepine	0.25-0.5	no
clonazepam	Klonopin	benzodiazepine	0.5-2	no
diazepam	Valium	benzodiazepine	2-10	no
estazolam	ProSom	benzodiazepine	1-2	yes
flurazepam	Dalmane	benzodiazepine	15-30	yes
lorazepam	Ativan	benzodiazepine	1-4	no
quazepam	Doral	benzodiazepine	7.5-15	yes
temazepam	Restoril	benzodiazepine	7.5-30	yes
triazolam	Halcion	benzodiazepine	0.125-0.25	yes
zaleplon	Sonata	nonbenzodiazepine	5-10	yes

eszopiclone	Lunesta	nonbenzodiazepine	1-3	yes
zolpidem	Ambien	nonbenzodiazepine	5-10	yes
zolpidem ER	Ambien CR	nonbenzodiazepine	6.25-12.5	yes
ramelteon	Rozerem	selective melatonin receptor agonist	8	yes
amitriptyline	Elavil	antidepressant	10-25	no
doxepin	Sinequan	antidepressant	10-70	no
mirtazapine	Remeron	antidepressant	15-30	no
nefazodone	Serzone	antidepressant	100	no
trazodone	Desyrel	antidepressant	50-300	no

HOW SLEEPING MEDICATIONS CREATE PROBLEMS

Sleeping medications can affect the way you feel and act during the day, negatively impacting your mood and impairing your ability to perform normal tasks throughout the day. They can also change your sleep cycle and the quality of your sleep. Knowing the ways that sedative-hypnotics can affect your overall life and potentially create problems is important for making a truly informed decision about whether to take them, or whether to continue taking them if you already are.

During the Day

Sleeping medications can affect your daytime functioning and performance, and not in a positive way. Since some amount of the sleeping medication may remain in your body the next day, it only makes sense that you may have some residual effects. Not only can they leave you feeling more sleepy and fatigued the next day, studies have also found that the use of certain sedative-hypnotics can result in decreased psychomotor and cognitive performance (Hindmarch et al. 2006). In other words, you may experience slower reaction time, impaired coordination, and even short-term amnesia or memory problems (Millar et al. 2007). This means you'll need to avoid driving or operating machinery or exercise caution when doing so, as you may still be somewhat drowsy from the medication. Sleeping medications also bring an increased risk of accidents, including motor vehicle crashes (Glass et al. 2005).

In addition, you may be more likely to slip or fall (Leipzig, Cumming, and Tinetti 1999), as sedative-hypnotics can cause dizziness and loss of balance. Even over-the-counter sleeping aids can cause you to feel drowsy and fatigued the next day, thus affecting your ability to perform a variety of tasks. So don't believe that enhanced sleep will help you function better the day after taking a sedative-hypnotic, because the evidence just doesn't support that notion. In fact, they won't even necessarily enhance your sleep.

While Sleeping

Sleeping pills can also cause problems during sleep. They affect respiration, often slowing it down, which can be a problem if you snore or have sleep apnea or other respiratory problems. If you have sleep apnea, you should be very cautious about using sedative-hypnotics, as they can worsen your respiratory events, causing the cessations or pauses in your breathing to last longer and occur more frequently. This, in turn, can increase your risk for heart and lung dysfunction (Spielman and Anderson 1999).

The majority of sedative-hypnotics also affect your sleep in another way: They alter your sleep architecture, changing the amount of time you spend in each stage of sleep. Benzodiazepines, for example, are known to increase stage N2 sleep, while suppressing or decreasing stage N3, or delta, sleep. Since delta sleep is the solid, deep sleep thought to be the most restorative part of the sleep cycle, having less of it can affect the overall quality of your sleep and how refreshed you feel upon arising. Some sedative-hypnotics may also decrease REM sleep, another important part of your sleep cycle (Morin 1993). As mentioned above, some of the newer nonbenzodiazepine drugs seem to have less impact on sleep architecture.

WHEN AND HOW TO STOP TAKING SLEEP MEDICATIONS

The decision to stop taking sleeping medications is a big one. Although nonpharmacological solutions generally offer better long-term results, learning and implementing these techniques can be more time-consuming than just taking a pill, and these approaches require a commitment on your part. However, there are many reasons why you may want to stop taking sedatives. Perhaps you're tired of having to take sleeping pills every night or worried about the effects of these drugs on your brain and body. Perhaps you're fed up with the idea that you'll need to take sleeping pills for the rest of your life in order to sleep well, or maybe the cost of the medications is taking a bite out of your wallet. Perhaps you don't like the idea of being reliant on medications and just want to see if you can sleep well on your own, without the help of sleeping pills.

There are also a few reasons why you may consider it worthwhile to take sleep medications. For example, if you take antihistamines because you have severe nasal allergies that are accompanied by insomnia, you may choose to remain on your medications in order to treat these symptoms. Similarly, if you have anxiety that's unrelated to insomnia and are taking benzodiazepines for your anxiety, you may want to keep taking your medication if it's working well for you. It's a good idea to discuss these issues with your doctor. Some parasomnias (disruptive sleep-related disorders, the topic of chapter 11), such as sleepwalking and sleep terrors, are also treated with benzodiazepines. If this is the case for you, it may be difficult for you to stop taking your medication because your parasomnia symptoms may reappear.

You'll need to weigh all of these factors carefully before making a decision about whether and when to stop taking sleeping pills. The rest of this chapter will provide you with the information you need to make the decision that's right for you. If you do decide to stop, it's a good idea to find the right time to do so, and to determine whether you need medical guidance or supervision during the process. You should be aware of the possible side effects of stopping too quickly, as well as the likely reactions that your body will have on the first night without medications.

Potential Side Effects of Stopping Sleep Medications

If you stop taking sleeping medications cold turkey, you have a higher likelihood of experiencing some type of withdrawal effect. The severity and duration of the symptoms is dependent on how long you've been taking sleeping pills, how often you take them, and the dosage you take. It's also dependent on the type of sleeping pills. Benzodiazepines generally cause more withdrawal effects than nonbenzodiazepines, but you can have problems when discontinuing either type of medication rapidly. With benzodiazepines, you may have seizures during withdrawal, so a careful, gradual stepping down from higher to lower doses is a better method than going cold turkey or ramping down your use quickly.

Possible effects of withdrawal from benzodiazepines include anxiety, irritability, headaches, fatigue, muscle tremors, rebound insomnia, and nausea; in addition, your senses can be heightened (Morin 1993). Rapid withdrawal from other sedative-hypnotics can cause rebound insomnia, heightened anxiety, behavioral changes, abdominal and muscle cramps, nausea, vomiting, sweating, increased heart rate, tremors, and seizures. You should seek medical attention if your symptoms are severe. Rebound insomnia accompanied by anxiety can be one of the most frustrating and disturbing symptoms when coming off of sedative-hypnotics, but it's only a short-term problem, and in the long run, your future without sleeping pills won't be so bleak. This is just a normal and temporary reaction to stopping most types of sleeping medications.

Although gradually titrating or lowering your dosage down can help lessen the extent of rebound insomnia, you should be prepared for the possibility that it will occur. Rebound insomnia is one of the biggest reasons why people continue to take sleeping pills, even when the medication doesn't work as well as when they first started taking it. In addition, rebound insomnia can actually be worse than your insomnia was before you started taking sleeping pills, and it can be accompanied by significant anxiety. The result is that you may be tempted to start taking sleeping pills again, just to avoid the rebound insomnia. Unfortunately, this actually reinforces the belief that you can't sleep without medications, thereby increasing your psychological dependence. As difficult as it may be, one of the most effective ways to overcome this faulty belief is to stick it out and not pop another sleeping pill.

Once you've gotten through the bad nights of rebound insomnia, you will have overcome one of the worst parts of stopping sleeping medications. It only makes sense that you'd experience more insomnia after stopping sedative-hypnotics. Even if you didn't feel your sleep medication was working very well for you, it was, in fact, having a sedative effect on your brain. Understanding that rebound insomnia is normal and that it won't last forever will help you get through one of the most difficult challenges in this sleep program: forgoing sleeping medications and giving your body a chance to fall asleep without pills.

Assessing Your Need for Medical Guidance or Supervision

To know whether you need medical supervision and guidance as you stop taking sedative-hypnotics, let's go through a few questions about your body's level of dependence on sleeping pills.

___ yes	___ no	1. Do you take sleeping pills every night?
___ yes	___ no	2. Do you take a higher dosage than prescribed?

___ yes	___ no	3. Have you ever had a bad reaction when you didn't take your sleep medication, or when trying to stop taking it? (For example, hot sweats, chills, rapid heart beat, seizures, or very bad insomnia.)
___ yes	___ no	4. Have you been taking sleeping pills five to seven nights per week for more than three months?

If you answered yes to any of these questions, you should consult with your doctor before you stop taking your sleeping pills so that you can be properly monitored for any possible negative reactions. Let's take a closer look at each question and what your answers mean.

If you answered yes to question 1, you may have developed either physical or psychological dependence on the medication. You may also fear rebound insomnia, a common reaction to discontinuing sleeping medications that reflects your body's physical dependence on sleeping pills. Rebound insomnia is a typical reaction when discontinuing sleeping medications, but it doesn't last forever. It may occur just the first night, or it may go on for several nights or even a few weeks. Although you may feel frustrated by rebound insomnia, the trick is to remember that your body needs some time to adjust to getting to sleep without the drug. While rebound insomnia may make you want to start taking sleeping pills again, it's better to stick it out for a few nights so your body loses its dependence on the drug.

If you answered yes to question 2, you've developed physical tolerance to your sleeping medication. For example, if you took 10 mg of Ambien for several months but then found it wasn't working for you anymore and started taking 20 mg each night, you've developed tolerance to the drug. This is a sign that you definitely need medical guidance and supervision to taper off the medication, as your body may have significant adverse reactions.

If you answered yes to question 3, you've already had an adverse reaction to trying to stop taking sleeping pills, a sign that your body is physically dependent on the drug. It's important that you discuss this with your doctor so you can taper off the medication in the way that's safest for you. Withdrawing from sedative-hypnotics can cause serious side effects in the body, just like withdrawing from alcohol and other addictive drugs. Depending on which medication you've been taking, the side effects can be significant.

If you answered yes to question 4, you've been taking sleeping pills for quite some time. It's possible that you're physically dependent on the medication, and very likely that you're psychologically dependent on it. The psychological hurdle can be one of the hardest to overcome, but the reality is that the vast majority of people can learn to sleep without the use of medications, so why not give yourself a chance to do so? It may be harder for you if you've been taking sleeping pills for a long time, because you've probably convinced yourself over time that sleeping pills are a necessity for you. But even chronic insomniacs who have used medication for years on end have successfully stopped taking sleeping pills.

Even if you answered no to all of the questions above, it's still important to assess whether you are physically or psychologically dependent on sleeping pills. Do you believe that you can't fall asleep without medications? Do you sometimes try to start falling asleep without medications but after a while simply give in and take sleeping pills anyway? If you answered yes to either of these questions, you may be psychologically dependent on sleeping drugs. This book can help you to work through psychological dependence on sleeping medications. Even if your dependence is only psychological and not physical, it's never a bad idea to let your doctor know that you'll be trying a new sleep program that doesn't involve medications.

Practical Tips for Stopping Sleeping Pills

If you decide you're ready to stop taking sleep medications, here are some helpful tips on how to go about it. If you haven't been using sleeping medications for a very long time or if you use them only rarely, certain aspects of this list won't apply to you. For example, you probably don't need to worry about rebound insomnia or slowly tapering off of your medication if you take it only on rare occasions. However, if you do take sleeping pills nearly every night, then all of these tips should be helpful:

- Consult with your doctor about the best way to taper down or decrease your dose. Since sleeping medications differ significantly in dosages, it's a good idea to get a medication taper schedule from your doctor. For some pills you may cut the dose in half initially, and for others you may take one-fourth of the dose. Each week, you would continue to cut the dosage down by the same proportion.

- Set a schedule for when you'll taper off of your sleeping pills. This should be a time when you aren't overly stressed, such as over the weekend or during a week when your workload isn't very heavy. There may never be a perfect time to stop, because life always entails some amount of stress; just try to pick a time when you think you won't be bombarded by too many other obligations or stressful or difficult events.

- Garner support from family and friends. Talk to them about how and why you want to stop taking sleeping medications once and for all. You may need to explain the negative impacts these medications are having on you and your life.

- Be prepared for rebound insomnia. Remember that it's a normal reaction your body is likely to have when coming off of sleeping pills. Rather than feeling overly anxious or frustrated by a few sleepless nights, try to find some peace of mind in knowing that this is the biggest hurdle to learning to sleep on your own.

- Practice relaxation exercises (see chapter 5) to prepare for the process of stopping the medication. Practicing in advance ensures you'll be skilled at using these techniques when you stop taking sleep medications.

- Once you've tapered down to the point where you aren't taking your sleep medication anymore, throw out your remaining pills. This is especially important if you were taking them on a nightly basis. You don't want to start that habit again, so why tempt yourself by keeping the pills around?

- Stick with it! Discontinuing your use of sleeping pills is a major accomplishment and a testament to your willpower and strength. Only after you quit taking these drugs can you learn to sleep on your own.

One question you may have is *when* during this sleep program you should stop taking sleep medications. That depends on you and how much you believe in your own ability to sleep without medications. Ideally, you'd stop taking sleeping medications before starting this program, as you'll benefit considerably from knowing that you can complete this program and overcome your sleep problem without taking medication. But it is a physical and emotional challenge, and you can also decide to stop taking sleeping pills later in the program. To the best of your ability, do it earlier rather than later. Remember, the goal of this program is to achieve a good night's sleep in a natural way—without medications. Learning that you are in control of your own sleep and can achieve restful sleep without drugs will reinforce that goal and help you maintain long-lasting results.

SUMMING UP

We live in a drug culture. Over-the-counter and prescription medications are taken for practically every minor symptom we experience, including our moods and, of course, insomnia. Herbal remedies are also very popular, particularly for sleep. While these options may be tempting, they don't treat the root of the problem, so you'll probably find yourself back where you started if you decide to stop taking sleep aids. And because sleeping pills can affect your sleep architecture, they may actually exacerbate your sleep problem. In addition, they can impair your daytime functioning, and regular use of sedative-hypnotics often leads to dependency. Although sleep aids can be helpful on a short-term basis when you're experiencing excessive stress, they aren't a good long-term solution. Fortunately, you can learn drug-free ways to sleep better at night, and this book will show you how. It's a tough challenge, but well worth it in the end.

As you read forward, chapters 4 through 10 require active participation on your part. This will mean focusing on, and probably changing, some of your behaviors. For example, learning new ways to handle stress and other factors that cause insomnia may require making important behavioral changes. In addition, this approach will ask you to examine your thinking patterns and change them if they're disrupting your sleep.

CHAPTER 4

Sleep Hygiene

Katie is a forty-five-year-old woman who has both sleep onset insomnia and sleep maintenance insomnia, so she has trouble both falling asleep and staying asleep. She describes her sleep problem as very frustrating, because she doesn't think she's particularly anxious or worried about anything. In fact, she said the only thing she's worried about is not falling asleep. Her sleeping problems began last year when she was taking care of her elderly father who had been diagnosed with cancer. This was a very difficult time for her, and her sleep schedule was quite erratic. At times, she needed to assist her father in the middle of the night, and she says that she's been a much lighter sleeper since that time. Although her father passed away six months ago, Katie's sleeping problems continue. When she gets into bed at night, she feels wide awake and has trouble turning off her mind. She says she's not particularly worried, she just starts thinking about things she has to do the next day and other topics that don't feel very stressful to her. She does, however, spend a lot of time thinking about how long it will take her to fall asleep that night. In fact, she's so concerned about her sleep that she finds herself thinking about it throughout the day, as well.

Katie tries to maintain a healthy lifestyle. She has one cup of coffee in the morning and sometimes another cup at lunchtime. She exercises several evenings each week at around 7 p.m. and has dinner around 8 p.m. She enjoys chocolate and usually has a few pieces after dinner each night. When her father became sick, she started smoking cigarettes, something she hadn't done since her college years. However, she has since cut back to a couple of cigarettes per day and is hopeful that she can quit soon. She typically has one glass of wine at night on weeknights, but has three or four drinks if she goes out with friends on the weekend.

Katie typically gets into bed at 10 p.m. even though she doesn't feel sleepy then. Katie explains, "I know it's going to take me such a long time to fall asleep at night that I want to give myself extra time in bed each night." Sometimes she watches TV or reads in bed while trying to relax, but neither helps her fall asleep more easily. During the night, she watches the clock while tossing and turning and feels increasingly frustrated with each passing minute. Sometimes it takes her over two hours to fall asleep. On a good night, she lies in bed feeling restless for at least *forty-five minutes before falling asleep. But she says a good night only happens about once or twice per month. She tried taking sleeping pills after her father passed away, and the medication worked great initially, allowing her to fall asleep within twenty minutes and to sleep for about seven hours straight each night. But gradually she needed higher and higher doses and started taking it every night, rather than one or two times per week, as prescribed, and the positive effects of the medication still continued to diminish. Now the medication doesn't work for Katie anymore, and rather than start taking a new medication, she wants to solve her sleep problem without medication.*

Katie says she typically wakes up three or four times at night and has trouble falling back asleep. She isn't sure what wakes her up. Sometimes she has to use the bathroom, but she doesn't think this is what's waking her. She feels wide awake during these nighttime awakenings and, depending on the time of night, either stays in bed trying to go back to sleep or just gets up and starts her day. If she finds herself lying in bed for over an hour without being able to get back to sleep, sometimes she gets out of bed and does some work on her computer. Katie works from home and keeps her computer and desk in her bedroom. She says it's easy for her to switch gears and just start working if she feels too frustrated to sleep.

Nighttime is frustrating for a lot of people. Katie is a typical example of someone with both sleep onset insomnia (trouble falling asleep) and sleep maintenance insomnia (trouble staying asleep). In fact, many of Katie's habits actually contribute to her sleep problem. Although you may not realize it, there's a good chance that many of your behaviors are likewise making your sleep problem worse. Fortunately, there are a number of simple ways to improve the likelihood that you'll get a good night of sleep. These include good sleep hygiene, which is the foundation of good sleep—and often one of the easiest and most straightforward strategies to implement.

Although many people are aware of the importance of maintaining their physical and mental health through exercise, good diet, regular medical check-ups, stress reduction techniques, and so on, they often forget that sleep is an essential component of both physical and mental well-being. However, lack of sleep or poor sleep can cause health problems and affect your mind and mood. In this chapter, we'll look at how you can improve your sleep by improving your *sleep hygiene*, which is simply the behaviors, conditions, and practices that surround sleep. In good sleep hygiene, these behaviors, conditions, and practices promote continuous, restful, effective sleep. While good sleep hygiene is important for everyone, it's especially important for those who have trouble sleeping. Good sleep hygiene can help you sleep better each night, which in turn can improve your overall health and well-being. The rest of this chapter discusses different aspects of sleep hygiene and offers suggestions about how you can improve your sleep-promoting behaviors.

LIMIT THE TIME YOU SPEND IN BED

Katie could improve many aspects of her sleep hygiene. For example, it's important to engage in relaxing, sleep-promoting activities as bedtime approaches, and to not get into bed until you're really feeling sleepy. Katie often gets into bed before she feels sleepy because she wants to give herself extra time to fall asleep. Although many people with insomnia do the same thing, it actually ends up making insomnia worse. If you spend time in bed when you're wide awake and not ready to fall asleep, you condition your body to feel wide awake whenever you get into bed. Many people fall into this trap.

Similarly, people who have trouble sleeping often start to worry about the total number of hours they sleep each night. So they get into bed earlier than their typical bedtime in the hopes that somehow they will manage to get more sleep throughout the night. However, it typically ends up working against them, and this leads to more frustration and difficulty with falling asleep. It can become a vicious cycle, so it's important that you get into bed only when you feel very sleepy.

On the same note, if you wake up during the night and have trouble falling back asleep, you should get out of bed and do something relaxing or boring in another room until you feel sleepy again. It's important that you don't lie awake in bed for a long time, and that you don't engage in stimulating activities in bed. Again, doing so will cause you to associate your bed with wakefulness, not sleep.

DON'T READ OR WATCH TV IN BED

Katie watches television or reads in bed each night before going to sleep. Unfortunately, these activities are making her insomnia worse. You may wonder how that's possible, when so many people watch TV or read in bed on a regular basis. In fact, you may remember a time when you did these things and still slept well. Watching TV and reading in bed are fine if you sleep well and don't have any trouble falling asleep. But if you do have problems sleeping, these activities are likely to make your situation worse. This is true for other activities too, such as eating, writing, talking on the phone, or using your laptop in bed. As with getting into bed too early, engaging in stimulating activities in bed trains your body to think it's okay to feel wide awake when you're in bed. It's best to read and watch television in the living room or another area of the house other than the bedroom.

Your bed should be reserved for sleep and sex only. Depending on the person, sex can be a stimulating activity that makes it more difficult to fall asleep or one that is very relaxing and makes it easier to fall asleep. If you fall into the first category and feel wide awake after sex, you may want to try having sex at other times of day or at least earlier in the evening. That way, it may be less likely to disrupt your sleep. Similarly, if you feel comfortable having sex in rooms other than your bedroom, you may want to try that. This is a very individualized decision and only you can know what feels right and comfortable.

SO WHAT SHOULD YOU DO BEFORE BEDTIME?

So what should you do in those late evening hours before you start feeling sleepy? Try to engage in relaxing activities for at least an hour before bedtime. This means nothing too stimulating, such as working, answering e-mails, making telephone calls, or anything stressful. Instead, consider meditation, relaxation exercises, stretching or yoga, deep breathing, engaging in quiet conversation with a family member or friend, or taking a warm bath. You might also read a book, listen to music, or possibly watch TV—but not in your bedroom, and only if these aren't too stimulating. And if you choose to read or watch television before bed and continue having trouble sleeping, you should experiment with doing different activities before bed.

It's important to establish a nightly routine that's calming in nature, without the pressures and stress that your daytime hours may include. If you find it difficult to unwind and achieve a calm, relaxed state at the end of the day, you'll find it helpful to start practicing the relaxation exercises in chapter 5. They'll help you relax your muscles, breathe more deeply, and feel calm. Like so many other things in life, practice makes perfect, so the more you practice relaxing your mind and body, the better you'll be at it. Relaxation techniques are particularly helpful when you're having trouble sleeping due to feeling too wound up or on edge. They can help you relax and achieve the calm state necessary for falling asleep both in the evening hours before bedtime and also if you can't sleep in the middle of the night.

DON'T WATCH THE CLOCK!

Do you find yourself looking at the clock often during the night, like Katie does? This is a common behavior for people with insomnia, but a problematic one. Every time you look at the clock while you're trying to fall asleep, it sends a signal to your brain reminding you that you're still awake and now have even fewer hours available for sleep that night. As a result, your anxiety about falling asleep is likely to increase. Sometimes you may even find yourself thinking, "Uh-oh, now it's 2:30 a.m., and I'm still awake" or "Now I'll really be a wreck tomorrow." Turn the clock around or cover it up so that you can't see it. As simple as this may sound, it can help reduce some of your anxious thoughts.

WHAT ABOUT CAFFEINE?

What other things does Katie do that may disrupt her sleep? Although the one cup of coffee in the morning is unlikely to have much effect on her nighttime sleep, she sometimes has another cup in the afternoon, and she eats chocolate each night after dinner. Although you may already be aware that caffeine can interfere with falling asleep, you should know that it can also cause you to wake up during the night, even if you don't have trouble falling asleep. Caffeine can take three to ten hours to be metabolized in your system, depending upon your age (Spielman and Anderson 1999). So caffeine could actually be waking you up during the night. In fact, many people still feel the effects of caffeine up to twelve hours after intake, so if you have trouble sleeping, it's a good idea to consume it only moderately, and to avoid it altogether after noon. It's important to be aware of how much caffeine you consume on a daily basis so you'll know if this might be a factor in your sleep problem. The next exercise will help you figure that out.

Assessing Your Caffeine Consumption

The following table lists the typical amount of caffeine in some common beverages, foods, and medications. For those of you who consume caffeine, indicate how many servings you typically have in the spaces provided, for before noon and after noon, and then calculate the number of milligrams (mg) of caffeine you typically consume before noon and after noon. Migraine and pain relief pills include

Anacin, Cafergot, Ercaf, Migergot, Cafgesic Forte, Combiflex, Excedrin, and Midol; allergy and cold remedies that contain caffeine include Coryban-D and Dristan; and over-the-counter stimulants that contain caffeine include NoDoz and Vivarin. Read the labels of any medications you take to determine whether they contain caffeine, and if so, how much. Add those amounts to your totals.

Products with caffeine	mg caffeine per serving	servings per day before noon	mg caffeine per day before noon	servings per day after noon	mg caffeine per day after noon
Coffee, brewed, 5 oz	60-180				
Coffee, instant, 5 oz	30-120				
Red Bull, 8.2 oz	80				
Sodas and colas, 12 oz	35-55				
Tea, black, 5 oz	30-65				
Tea, green or white, 8 oz	15-20				
Dark chocolate, 1 oz	20				
Baking chocolate, 1 oz	25-35				
Milk chocolate, 1 oz	6				
Iced tea, 12 oz	67-76				
Espresso, 2 oz	45-125				
Cappuccino, 8 oz	60				
Latte, 8 oz	60				
Hot cocoa, 8 oz	14-30				
Chocolate milk, 8 oz	5				
Decaf coffee, brewed, 5 oz	2-5				
Decaf coffee, instant, 5 oz	1-5				
Migraine and pain relief pills, 1 dose	40-130				
Allergy and cold remedies	25-30				
Over-the-counter stimulants	100-200				
TOTAL					

Source: Based on data from Curtis and Schuler 2004; Carlson 1998; and Ray and Ksir 1993.

Add up the amount of caffeine you typically consume each day before noon and after noon. For those with sleep problems, it's a good idea to avoid caffeine after noon and to limit morning intake to 100 to 200 mg. Caffeine sensitivity differs from person to person, but research indicates that consuming 200 mg of caffeine in the morning can affect sleep architecture (Landolt et al. 1995).

OTHER STIMULANTS THAT AFFECT SLEEP

What about other stimulants that may be affecting your sleep? Although many people associate smoking cigarettes with relaxation and a restful state of mind, nicotine is actually a stimulant. Katie's smoking is probably interfering with her sleep. If you smoke and haven't been able to quit, at least try to decrease the number of cigarettes you smoke in the evening, and don't smoke for an hour or so before bedtime. If you find it very difficult to go that long without smoking, at least decrease your nicotine consumption by only taking a couple of puffs on your cigarette and throwing the rest of it out. Some people with insomnia smoke in the middle of the night when they can't sleep. This will definitely make a sleep problem worse.

Other stimulants that may be affecting your sleep include herbs such as ginseng and ephedra and illicit drugs such as cocaine. Ecstasy (MDMA) can also have stimulant qualities because it is an amphetamine and because it may be laced with cocaine or other drugs. Research has found that food coloring can increase hyperactivity in children, so it may be advisable to watch your intake of products with food coloring, as well. As discussed in chapter 2, certain medications can also cause sleep disturbances, such as antidepressants, blood pressure medications, cholesterol medications, antiarrhythmic drugs, corticosteroids, bronchodilators, Parkinson's drugs, antiepileptic drugs, decongestants, stimulants, asthma medications, and thyroid medications (see chapter 2 for a listing of commonly prescribed drugs in these categories). It's important to ask your doctor and pharmacist about whether any of your medications interfere with sleep, and to read the information on medication side effects for all drugs that you take to determine whether medications may be causing your sleep problem or making it worse. Sometimes a combination of medications can cause insomnia. If you think this is part of the problem for you, be sure to discuss the issue with your doctor and pharmacist so you can find a solution that works for you.

HOW THE TIMING OF EXERCISE AFFECTS SLEEP

Exercise is important for your overall health and your sleep, so you should try to fit it into your schedule on a regular basis. However, the timing of exercise can impact your sleep due to its effects on your circadian rhythm and body temperature. As a reminder, circadian rhythm refers to the cycle, roughly twenty-four hours in length, of various physiological, behavioral, and biochemical processes. Circadian rhythms originate within the body, but they can be affected by environmental factors. Body temperature varies over a twenty-four-hour period, typically having two peaks and two troughs per cycle. You're most likely to fall asleep when your body temperature is dropping, or on the downward slope. This typically occurs during the early to midafternoon hours and again at night. However, exercise increases your body temperature, so if you exercise too late in the day, it will take longer for your body temperature to drop.

The best time to exercise is about four to five hours before bedtime. If you aren't able to exercise then, exercising in the morning is also fine. Exercising in the hours close to bedtime, however, can disrupt your sleep. If you exercise after work, try to do so right away, rather than waiting until later in the evening.

HOW EXPOSURE TO LIGHT AFFECTS SLEEP

Light is one of the primary external factors exerting an influence on circadian rhythms, and the amount of exposure you have to light each day can definitely affect your sleep. This includes both sunlight and artificial lighting. Our brains naturally produce melatonin, a sleep-promoting hormone, when it's dark. If you're exposed to bright light in the evening hours or if you have significant exposure to sunlight in the afternoon and early evening hours, it can decrease or delay your production of melatonin. The answer is *not* to simply take melatonin supplements, though that may seem tempting, especially since it's readily available over the counter. But remember, supplemental melatonin isn't regulated by the FDA, nor has it been proven effective for insomnia. So rather than taking supplements, you want to alter your environment so your brain produces melatonin naturally in response to darkness. Let's take a look at how this works with sleep disorders related to a disrupted circadian rhythm: delayed sleep phase disorder and advanced sleep phase disorder.

Delayed Sleep Phase Disorder

If you find that you can't fall asleep until very late at night but then sleep straight through the night and have difficulty waking up until later in the morning, you may have delayed sleep phase disorder. Part of the treatment for this disorder, which typically presents itself as sleep onset insomnia, is to limit your exposure to light in the afternoon and evening hours, even if that means wearing sunglasses inside. It's also helpful to increase your exposure to light in the morning hours. This allows you to naturally reset your biological clock, or circadian rhythm.

In addition to adjusting your exposure to light throughout the day, you should set your alarm clock for the same time each morning, including on the weekends, and be sure to wake up and get out of bed when the alarm goes off. Try to go to bed fifteen minutes earlier than your usual bedtime. Once you're able to fall asleep at that time for one solid week, move your bedtime forward by fifteen minutes once again. This allows you to shift your biological clock gradually. There's also a more rapid method. This involves staying up all night and not allowing yourself to fall asleep the next day. Wait until your ideal bedtime to go to bed the following night. You'll be so sleep deprived that you shouldn't have much trouble falling asleep. If you use this faster method, it's crucial to maintain your new schedule, getting up at the same time each morning. If you choose to try the faster method, don't drive or operate machinery after you've stayed up all night, as sleep deprivation can impair your performance and make these activities dangerous.

Advanced Sleep Phase Disorder

If you find yourself falling asleep earlier in the evening than your ideal bedtime, like 7 or 8 p.m., and then waking up at 3 or 4 a.m. unable to get back to sleep, you could have advanced sleep phase disorder. When you calculate the number of hours you sleep at night, it's probably between seven and eight hours, so lack of sleep isn't the problem, timing is; you're waking up too early in the morning, when everyone else is still sleeping. If you think you have advanced sleep phase disorder, the solution is opposite that for delayed sleep phase disorder: You need to expose yourself to more bright light in the afternoon and evening hours, and to stay active and busy in the evenings. Try going out to dinner, inviting friends over for the evening, or engaging in stimulating or fun activities like playing games. Taking a walk after dinner would also be a much better choice than sedentary activities like sitting and reading a book or watching TV in the evenings, where you might fall asleep.

Since it can be hard to keep yourself awake when you're very tired, try to change your bedtime gradually. For example, for the first week, set your bedtime twenty to thirty minutes later than usual. Once you've done that for a week, once again adjust your bedtime twenty to thirty minutes later the next week. Follow that schedule until you've established a regular bedtime that's optimal for you. As you gradually shift your circadian rhythm, you should start sleeping later. This is especially true if you weren't having frequent awakenings before, but simply fell asleep too early and woke up too early. It's important to stick to your new sleep schedule. You may also find it helpful to wear sunglasses and limit your exposure to bright light in the morning—the opposite of the approach used for delayed sleep phase disorder.

HOW ALCOHOL AFFECTS SLEEP

Many people ask if having a glass of wine or a beer will help them fall asleep. According to a study that looked at the economic impact of insomnia, Americans spend over $780 million per year on alcohol in attempts to combat their insomnia (Walsh and Engelhardt 1999). In another study, 13 percent of eighteen- to forty-five-year-olds in the general population reported using alcohol in the past year to aid in sleep (Gillin and Drummond 2000). However, in spite of how common this practice is, drinking alcohol definitely isn't the answer to your sleep problem.

Alcohol affects sleep in different ways. Although you may find that you fall asleep more easily after having a couple of drinks in the evening, alcohol actually tends to disrupt sleep. It tends to increase NREM sleep and reduce REM sleep in the first hours after falling asleep. So you may sleep solidly for the first couple of hours, but because alcohol is metabolized rather quickly, you're likely to awaken more often during the latter two-thirds of your sleep period, as the alcohol leaves your system. In addition to waking up more often, you may spend more time in REM sleep, have nightmares, experience an increase in heart rate and sweating, and even have headaches, stomach problems, and a greater need to urinate (Gillin and Drummond 2000).

This may or may not be the case for you, but the next time you have a few drinks before bed, check and see if your night of sleep was as restful as you'd hoped it would be. Most likely, you woke up several times or just had an overall feeling of restlessness. After drinking, sleep is generally less restorative and can leave you more tired the next day. Although some people with insomnia try to self-medicate themselves with alcohol, it certainly isn't an effective solution to sleepless nights. Drugs such as marijuana, heroin, barbiturates, and, of course, cocaine and other stimulants can also negatively affect your sleep.

SET A REGULAR SLEEP SCHEDULE AND STICK TO IT

Another important component of improving your sleep is setting a regular time for going to bed and getting up and sticking to it! Although your bedtime may fluctuate a bit from time to time, especially on the weekends, it's important that you try to keep your schedule as regular as possible. Always aim for going to bed within one hour of your usual bedtime, whether earlier or later. For example, if you usually go to bed at 10 p.m., avoid going to bed any earlier than 9 p.m. or any later than 11 p.m. Larger deviations can really throw your sleep schedule off. If you do end up going to bed much later than usual one night, you should still try to wake up at your usual time the next morning. If not, you're likely to have trouble falling asleep the next night.

Also, if you're having trouble with insomnia, it isn't a good idea to take naps during the day. You only need a certain number of hours of sleep over a twenty-four-hour period, and naps count toward that total. If you take a one- or two-hour nap during the day, you'll likely have more trouble falling asleep that night, as your body has already gotten some extra sleep.

FORGET ABOUT A MAGIC NUMBER OF HOURS OF SLEEP

Most people believe they need a certain number of hours of sleep each night. We've all heard statements about the importance of getting at least seven or eight hours of sleep per night for health and well-being. However, these numbers are just averages across huge populations. As discussed in chapter 1, some people are short sleepers and others long sleepers. Many people sleep less than seven hours nightly on a regular basis and still function perfectly well and feel fine during the day. I've heard some people say that as long as they can get a solid four hours of sleep, they feel great during the day. On the other hand, some people don't feel refreshed unless they get nine or ten hours of sleep each night. It's totally variable, and not something you should be concerned about. Try to think back to before your sleep was a problem. If you typically slept about six hours per night and felt fine, then there's no need for you to try to achieve some number that's unrealistic for you. One of the most important things you can do is stop focusing so much time and attention on getting a certain number of hours of sleep each night and instead focus on how you feel during the day after a good night of sleep versus a bad night of sleep. Then compare the number of hours you actually slept each night to get a better idea of how much sleep your body actually needs.

Assessing How Much Sleep Is Right for You

For one week, keep track of how many hours you sleep at night and how you feel the next day. This will give you a better idea of your personal sleep requirements. When you assess how you feel the next morning, and then during the rest of the day, consider whether you feel refreshed or tired, and how you feel generally: great, good, fair, or poor.

Date	Hours of sleep the previous night	How do you feel in the morning?	How do you feel during the rest of the day?

Hopefully this log helped you identify the amount of sleep that's right for you. If you still aren't sure, continue keeping this sort of log until you have a better idea how many hours of sleep you need each night. (Chapter 7 will also help you determine how much sleep you need.) As you work through the rest of this book, this is the amount of sleep you should aim for, not an arbitrary number based on averages.

IMPROVE YOUR SLEEP ENVIRONMENT

Your sleep environment is very important. Make sure that your bedroom is dark and quiet. If you're having trouble sleeping, the last thing you need is environmental stimuli, such as outside noises or lights peeking through your curtains, interfering with your sleep as well. Room temperature can also affect your sleep. You'll fall asleep easier and be more likely to stay asleep when the room is a comfortable temperature. Studies have shown that an ideal sleeping environment is neither too hot nor too cold (Glotzbach and Heller 2000; Roehrs, Zorick, and Roth 2000). Likewise, it's important to sleep on a mattress that's comfortable for you. People's preferences in mattresses and how well they sleep on different surfaces vary widely, so it isn't a matter of choosing a particular model or style. Instead, try to find a mattress that's comfortable for you, and consider replacing your current mattress if it's old and no longer offers good support.

In addition to these obvious environmental factors, other aspects of your sleeping situation can also play a role in how well you sleep. For example, Katie has her computer and desk in her bedroom and says that she can easily switch gears from trying to fall asleep to working. Many people who work from home find it difficult to separate their work from the rest of their lives. If you work from home, it's important that your office not be in your bedroom. Otherwise it's far too easy to work or think about working at night, rather than engaging in sleep-promoting activities. Plus, those who work from home typically spend many more hours doing work-related activities than they would if they went somewhere else to work each day. It's important to give yourself the time and space you need to relax and wind down, rather than going straight from work mode to sleep mode. Having a separate room for your office is important, and ideally you should shut the door of your home office each day to signal the end of your workday. Checking your e-mail and listening to voicemail can wait until the next day; don't engage in these or other work activities right before bedtime or in the middle of the night.

If your sleep partner stays up later than you, try to minimize household noise. For example, if your partner watches TV at night, ask your partner to wear headphones or watch TV in a room far enough from your bedroom that the noise won't disturb you. Ideally, your partner shouldn't be watching TV in your bedroom, as this can be distracting to you and make it harder to fall asleep. Similarly, if people in your house are playing video games, listening to music, or doing other activities that may disturb you at night, try to find an alternative time for them to do these things or at least have them do these activities in a part of the house where you won't be disturbed. If your partner snores, try wearing earplugs. This may help for other environmental noises as well. Similarly, putting a white noise machine in your bedroom can decrease the likelihood that you'll be disturbed by ambient noise in your home. If your partner gets into bed later than you, it's important that the room remain dark and that your partner doesn't make much noise in the room while getting ready for bed.

Sleep Hygiene Questionnaire

Now that you have a good understanding of sleep hygiene, you can assess your own sleep behavior, environment, and habits to determine whether you might make some changes that could help you sleep better.

____ yes	____ no	1. Do you lie in bed for hours, even when you aren't asleep?
____ yes	____ no	2. Do you read in bed?
____ yes	____ no	3. Do you watch television in bed?
____ yes	____ no	4. Do you eat, talk on the phone, or do other activities in bed?
____ yes	____ no	5. Do you engage in stimulating activities before bedtime?
____ yes	____ no	6. Do you watch the clock at night?
____ yes	____ no	7. Do you consume large quantities of caffeine, or consume any within twelve hours of bedtime?

___ yes	___ no	8. Do you smoke, either during the day or at night?
___ yes	___ no	9. Do you exercise within four hours of bedtime?
___ yes	___ no	10. Do you keep bright lights on until it's time for bed?
___ yes	___ no	11. Do you drink alcohol to help you sleep?
___ yes	___ no	12. Does your bedtime or wake up time often vary by more than an hour?
___ yes	___ no	13. Do you spend more time in bed on the weekends?
___ yes	___ no	14. Is your sleeping environment uncomfortable in any way?

If you answered yes to any of these questions, you need to improve certain aspects of your sleep hygiene. Let's look at each question in detail.

If you answered yes to question 1, you're conditioning yourself to associate your bed with wakefulness, which will make it difficult for you to sleep well! If you answered no, you're on the right track to breaking any associations you may have with your bed being a place where you don't sleep well.

If you answered yes to question 2, 3, or 4, you're engaging in stimulating activities while in bed. Please remember that the bed is for sleep and sex only. Watching television, reading books, talking on the phone, and other stimulating activities should take place in another room. If you answered no, you're on the right track with eliminating stimulating activities in bed.

If you answered yes to question 5, you need to try to relax before bedtime. This is very important in setting the stage for a restful night's sleep. If you answered no, then good job on realizing the importance of relaxation as part of your bedtime routine.

If you answered yes to question 6, remember this: Every time you look at the clock, you're just reminding yourself that you're still awake! This is likely to increase your anxiety and frustration, and that isn't restful. If you answered no, you probably already know how watching the clock can increase your anxiety about not sleeping.

If you answered yes to question 7, you're consuming too much caffeine, or your caffeine consumption occurs too close to bedtime. Some people are sensitive to the effects of caffeine for up to twelve hours, so experiment with avoiding caffeine for at least twelve hours before bedtime. If you answered no, continue to monitor your caffeine consumption and keep up the good work!

If you answered yes to question 8, you're decreasing your chances of getting a good night's sleep. Nicotine is a stimulant and can keep you awake. At a bare minimum, try to decrease the amount you smoke during the day, and especially at night. If possible, don't smoke for an hour before bedtime. If you answered no, then good job!

If you answered yes to question 9, you're exercising too late in the evening. The optimal time to exercise is four to five hours before bedtime. If that doesn't work with your schedule, then exercising even earlier in the day is better than exercising too close to bedtime. If you answered no, then you aren't disrupting your sleep by exercising too late in the evening.

If you answered yes to question 10, you're upsetting your circadian rhythm by stimulating your brain with light, which makes it harder for your body to realize that it's dark outside and time to sleep.

If you answered no, then continue to dim the lights at night as a way of helping your body prepare itself for sleep.

If you answered yes to question 11, you're making the mistake of using alcohol in an attempt to put yourself to sleep. Remember, although alcohol can make you feel sleepy initially, later in the night it disrupts your sleep and can actually cause you to wake up more often. If you answered no, you probably already know that alcohol isn't the answer to sleepless nights.

If you answered yes to question 12 or 13, your erratic sleep schedule could be contributing to your sleep problem. Try going to bed at the same time every night and getting up at the same time each morning, even on weekends. If you answered no, you're probably already aware of the importance of a consistent sleep-wake schedule.

If you answered yes to question 14, consider what changes you can make in your bedroom to improve your sleep environment. If you see street lights shining into your bedroom from outside, try using darker curtains or shades. If noise is an issue, you may want to experiment with earplugs or a white noise machine. The temperature in your room should also be comfortable for sleeping. If you answered no, then your sleeping environment is dark, quiet, and comfortable. You must already know how important it is to have a sleeping environment that helps promote sleep.

After realizing the importance of good sleep hygiene, Katie made some changes in her lifestyle and her behaviors leading up to bedtime. First of all, she cut out her cup of coffee at lunchtime and her chocolate after dinner. Although she initially found this difficult, she replaced her afternoon java with a quick walk around the block and found that her energy level actually increased in the afternoons. Once Katie realized that exercising late at night wasn't helpful, she began exercising earlier in the day. This also allowed her more time in the evenings to relax and wind down after working all day. Katie was also able to decrease her drinking. Although she still chose to have a few drinks with friends on occasion, she decided to do this only once a month, and if it disrupted her sleep, she understood why this was happening and didn't get anxious about it. Cutting down on cigarette smoking has been harder for Katie. Since she's physically addicted, she's having a hard time quitting. However, she has decreased the amount she smokes in the evenings and is usually able to abstain from smoking for the entire hour before bedtime. She's also sought the advice and support of her doctor and friends in an attempt to quit smoking soon.

A big change that Katie made was moving her office to another room in the house. She now restricts herself to working only in her separate office and doesn't work at night. If she wakes up during the night, she tries to do relaxing things rather than jumping back to work. Katie has improved her sleeping environment in other ways. She covered her clock in her room and said that she noticed a decrease in her level of anxiety about sleep from the very first night she did this. She also stopped reading and watching TV in bed and now does these activities in her living room. For the most part, Katie also only gets into bed when she feels sleepy, so she doesn't spend much time lying in bed while she feels wide awake. These changes have all improved Katie's sleep, and she feels that she's on the right track with regard to solving her sleep problem.

SUMMING UP

Maintaining good sleep hygiene is just one part of improving your sleep and overcoming insomnia, but it's a very important one. You may start sleeping better simply by following the good sleep practices outlined in this chapter. Although you may need to work on behavioral changes beyond simply improving your sleep hygiene, don't underestimate its importance. Anyone experiencing sleep problems will benefit from improving their sleep hygiene.

CHAPTER 5

Relaxation Techniques

Derrick always feels stressed-out. As a thirty-eight-year-old accountant, husband, and father of two small children, he feels like there's never enough time in the day. He works long hours and feels guilty about not being at home more. When he is at home, he tries to help his wife out as much as he can, but often ends up feeling overwhelmed and just turns on the TV for a few hours each night. He loves to spend time with his children, reading stories to them or playing games like hide-and-seek. When Derrick was younger, he was very athletic. Now he feels like he never has time to exercise and is about twenty pounds overweight. His job is stressful, and although he tries not to think about it when he gets home at night, he often jots down reminders to himself and even checks his work voicemail to make sure there are no problems he needs to handle. Before having children, Derrick and his wife used to regularly go out to dinner or meet up with friends. Now they tend to stay home most nights, and if they do go out, they bring their children along, which he doesn't find relaxing. Derrick is feeling burned-out and it's taking a toll on his physical and mental health. Not only has he gained weight, his blood pressure is up, and he's more irritable. And when he lies down to go to sleep at night, he feels like he can't shut off his mind. Sometimes he lies there for hours obsessing about problems at work and other stress in his life. Derrick isn't sure what to do next.

Learning to relax isn't easy for everyone. Like Derrick, most of us are running around from one place to the next all day long. Perhaps you're working, taking care of your kids, making dinner, doing laundry, keeping the house tidy, and trying to socialize with friends and spend time with family. Or perhaps you're a student, studying for exams, preparing for presentations, and trying to figure out what you want to do for the rest of your life. Or you may be retired, living on a fixed income, worrying about your health, trying to please your children and grandchildren, and feeling as though you aren't as free as you were when you were younger.

There just aren't enough hours in the day to do everything. So when it comes to taking time for relaxing, you may feel guilty for even sitting down when you think of all the other things you could be doing. You may find it difficult to justify "taking a break" when you look around and see how busy others are. But not finding time to relax can take a significant toll on you, both physically and mentally. Not only can it make it harder to deal with daily stress, it may also make it harder for you to wind down at the end of the day and get a good night of sleep.

The first step is to accept that relaxing is a good thing. Acknowledging that you need to relax in order to feel your best and be optimally productive each day is an important part of gaining more balance, and more control, over your life. So if you start feeling guilty when you try to relax, stop yourself! Remind yourself that everyone needs some downtime, and that taking time to relax each day can actually reenergize you and help you to feel better during the day and sleep better at night.

WHAT COUNTS AS RELAXING?

Although relaxing may seem like a straightforward concept, there's a lot of variation in what people find relaxing. You may find the very concept of relaxing frustrating because you're not sure where to begin. So let's start with a definition of the word "relax." Relax means to become less tense, less tight, less restrained; to rest, to become lax or loose, to relieve tension or strain. When you relax, your body, your mind, or both should feel the difference. So the question is, what kinds of activities do you like to do in order to relax? List your top five favorite relaxing activities here:

1. _____

2. _____

3. _____

4. _____

5. _____

Do the activities you listed help you relax both physically and mentally? Some activities help with just one or the other, and that's okay too, depending on the situation. Hopefully you've listed some that help physically and some that help mentally, so that you can choose a relaxing activity that's most appropriate to your situation at the time.

Relaxing Activities Checklist

Now that you've come up with some ideas on your own, let's explore other relaxing activities you might not have mentioned. Any of the activities listed below can help you relieve some stress in your life. Check off any of the following tension busters that appeal to you:

_____ Taking a bath

_____ Reading a book

_____ Riding a bike

_____ Going for a walk

_____ Listening to music

_____ Watching television

_____ Writing in your journal

_____ Playing a board game with family or friends

_____ Getting a manicure or pedicure

_____ Getting a massage

_____ Playing golf

_____ Swimming

_____ Knitting or sewing

_____ Gardening

_____ Watching a movie

_____ Going to the theater for a play, concert, or other performance

_____ Going out to dinner with friends or family

_____ Doing yoga

_____ Meditating

_____ Doing deep breathing exercises

_____ Playing with your pet

_____ Doing beading, ceramics, pottery, or other crafts

_____ Going to a park or the beach, or just being in nature

As you can see, this list could go on and on. Not all of these activities will be relaxing for everyone; for example, playing golf can be frustrating or stressful for some people, but relaxing for others. However, there are many to choose from, so experiment to find what works best for you and then incorporate those relaxing activities into your daily routine. It's good to have a variety of ways of relaxing that work well for you, because every day is different and some days you may need to do something different to relax.

When you're engaged in these activities, try to really focus on what you're doing at the time and let go of some of the stress you may carry around with you. If you do an activity one day that's mentally relaxing but requires you to do physical exercise, try a different activity another day that allows you to relax physically, as well. Making time for a relaxing activity every day may seem unrealistic to you at first, but once you start incorporating relaxation into your daily lifestyle, you'll begin to wonder how you ever managed without it!

SPECIFIC RELAXATION TECHNIQUES

While it's very important for you to integrate relaxing and enjoyable activities into your daily life, many people also benefit from specific relaxation exercises. The rest of this chapter will focus on some relaxation skills that may be new to you: diaphragmatic breathing, deep breathing, guided imagery, progressive muscle relaxation, and a technique that combines all of these skills. These exercises can help you relax by slowing down your breathing, creating calming mental images, or decreasing the tension in your muscles. Not everyone with insomnia has problems relaxing, but many people do, and all of us can benefit from learning to relax. So give each of these techniques a try to see if they can help you relax a bit more.

When doing any of these exercises, start by sitting upright in a comfortable chair. Your feet should be flat on the floor, with your arms resting comfortably at your sides. Closing your eyes may help you focus on the exercise. If you can't find a comfortable position while sitting upright, try reclining in a chair or on the couch or lying down. However, these relaxation exercises aren't intended to make you fall asleep; rather, they're meant to help you achieve a deeper level of relaxation so that when it's time for you to get into bed at night, you feel calmer and more at peace.

Breathing Exercises

For the following two breathing exercises, read through the entire exercise a few times before you try it so that you can remember the steps and do the exercise without having to read the instructions. Another option is to record the instructions and play the recording back to yourself each time you do the exercise until you've learned it.

Diaphragmatic Breathing

This exercise focuses on your breathing. Diaphragmatic breathing is a form of breathing that expands your abdomen or diaphragm, rather than your chest, as you inhale. The diaphragm is actually the primary breathing muscle in your body, but we often don't breathe this way due to the emphasis society places on a flat, toned abdomen. In addition, many people have tension in their back, chest, and stomach due to high stress levels. This can make it difficult for your diaphragm to perform the way it should: allowing the stomach to expand while breathing, rather than simply the chest.

To see how you're breathing, place one hand on your stomach, above your belly button but below your rib cage. Place your other hand on your chest. In diaphragmatic breathing, only the hand on your abdomen should move up and down when you breathe, while the hand on your chest remains essentially still. Diaphragmatic breathing allows you to breathe more efficiently, so it's less work for your muscles. It also allows you to keep your neck and shoulder muscles more relaxed while breathing (Poppen 1998).

Diaphragmatic breathing can have an overall calming effect, and since it's incompatible with shallow, rapid breathing, it can be especially helpful for reducing feelings of anxiety.

In addition to focusing on expanding your abdomen while breathing, make note of how many breaths you take each minute. Most people take between eight and twenty breaths per minute while at rest, with the average resting respiratory rate in healthy adults being about twelve breaths per minute (Sherwood 2006). While practicing diaphragmatic breathing, try to decrease your respiratory rate to about six breaths per minute. Slowing down your breathing will allow you to relax more and more with each breath you take. It's important to exhale slowly, as this will help you relax even more.

Now that you understand the overall concept, here's are some instructions for practicing diaphragmatic breathing. For this exercise, you need to have a clock close by so that you can measure your breathing rate. Sit in a comfortable chair with your feet flat on the floor. If you can't find a comfortable position while sitting upright, try reclining in a chair or even lying down the first few times you practice diaphragmatic breathing:

1. Place one hand on your abdomen and the other on your chest.

2. Take several slow, deep breaths through your nose.

3. Which of your hands is moving up and down? It should be the lower hand, the one on your abdomen. Your chest should remain relatively still during this breathing exercise.

4. Continue taking slow, deep breaths until you can feel your abdomen expanding and contracting with each breath you take.

5. Look at the clock and count how many breaths you take for one full minute.

6. Try to decrease the number of breaths you take to about six breaths per minute. If you inhale for about five seconds and exhale for about five seconds, your overall breathing rate will be about six breaths per minute. As a rough guide, slowly count 1-2-3-4-5 each time you inhale and 1-2-3-4-5 each time you exhale. If you prefer, you can say the letters A-B-C-D-E as you inhale and exhale.

7. Another way to slow down your breathing is to pause briefly after you inhale. So you inhale, counting 1-2-3-4-5 (or A-B-C-D-E), pause for a second or two, and then exhale for about five seconds.

8. If you can't initially inhale or exhale for a full five seconds, that's fine. Just start with what you can do, inhaling and exhaling for three or four seconds. With practice, your breathing will slow down and it will be easier for you to take regular, slow, deep breaths.

9. Keep a steady breathing pace. Once you can maintain a slow, even breathing pattern, close your eyes and repeat a soothing word in your head, such as "calm" or "peace," with each inhalation and exhalation.

Start off by practicing for just five minutes each day and work up to ten to fifteen minutes each day. Remember that practice makes perfect. For this breathing exercise to help you slow your breathing rate and decrease your level of anxiety when you're feeling stressed-out, upset, or tense, you need to already be good at it.

Deep Breathing

Now that you've learned how to do diaphragmatic breathing, you can move on to deep breathing. It's important to master diaphragmatic breathing first, because deep breathing incorporates parts of it. Deep breathing is just what it sounds like: very slow, deep breathing. It involves expanding the diaphragm and abdomen while inhaling, followed by expanding your chest. By involving the respiratory muscles of the chest in this deep breathing exercise, you're going one step further than you did with the diaphragmatic breathing. Of course, diaphragmatic breathing also fills your lungs with oxygen each time you inhale, but in diaphragmatic breathing you typically exhale before your chest also starts expanding, so only the hand on your abdomen moves up and down. With deep breathing, both hands move up and down.

You should still start off your breathing by inhaling slowly, allowing your abdomen to expand. Basically, you're pumping your lungs each time you expand your abdomen. This allows your lungs to fill up with oxygen without doing the pumping, which is what happens in shallow, rapid breathing. In this exercise, you'll take longer breaths than you did in diaphragmatic breathing, counting to ten with each inhalation and each exhalation. This exercise can be very powerful when you're feeling anxious or stressed. Now that you have a good understanding of the overall concept, here are some instructions for practicing deep breathing:

1. Sit in a comfortable chair.

2. Put one hand on your abdomen and the other hand on your chest.

3. Breathe in slowly and comfortably through your nose, then exhale through your nose, again slowly and comfortably. Continue breathing through your nose throughout the exercise.

4. Feel your abdomen rise and fall. Practice this for a few breaths.

5. Now slowly inhale again and then pause for a few seconds before exhaling. Your breathing should be very slow, even, and regular.

6. Slowly exhale.

7. Inhale slowly again and really feel how your abdomen expands and the air enters your lungs. The hand on your belly should rise, followed by a slight rise of the hand on your chest.

8. Slowly exhale, trying to keep your breathing as slow and even as you can.

9. Next, as you inhale, first expand your abdomen, then expand your chest to fill your lungs even further. Pause for a few seconds, and then slowly empty out the air, first from your chest area, then from your abdomen.

10. Next, try counting to ten with each breath. Inhale slowly, silently and slowly counting 1-2-3-4-5-6-7-8-9-10, then pause for one to three seconds, then release, exhaling and silently counting 1-2-3-4-5-6-7-8-9-10. If you prefer, you can also think of the letters A through J in your head as you inhale and exhale.

11. Your hands should remain on your abdomen and chest until you feel comfortable that you can do the exercise properly without them. At that point, feel free to rest your hands comfortably at your sides.

Initially, practice this deep breathing exercise for five minutes each day, and work up to ten to fifteen minutes each day if you like. Once you've gotten used to the slow-paced rhythm of this deep breathing exercise, you can repeat a soothing word such as "calm," "peace," or "breathe" in your head with each inhalation and exhalation.

Guided Imagery

The previous exercises focused on breathing. Now let's move on to guided imagery. This type of relaxation exercise involves imagining a certain place where you could feel very relaxed, such as the beach, a park, or a mountain. These exercises focus on the senses of sight, sound, smell, touch, and temperature to help you relax (Poppen 1998). By imagining a peaceful scene and then allowing yourself to become absorbed in the sensory experiences that go along with that imagined scene, you can achieve a significant level of calm and relaxation. While doing guided imagery, some people experience decreased tension, slower heart rate, deeper breathing, and a feeling of warmth in the hands and feet (Bourne 2005).

I've included several different scenes. Once you get the hang of guided imagery, you can create your own scenes tailored to what you find most relaxing. It's a good idea to read the scripts aloud and record them so you can play them back and practice them while keeping your eyes closed. Similarly, if you choose to create your own peaceful scenes, you can write them down first and then record them as you read them aloud. You can also buy a wide variety of relaxation and guided imagery CDs or download them from online music stores. The Resources section at the end of the book includes information on some recommended recordings that contain exercises similar to those in this chapter.

When recording visualization exercises, try to keep a slow, even pace as you read the script. This will help you maintain a calm and soothing tone throughout the exercise. Before you start the actual visualization, take a few slow breaths. Sit comfortably in a chair or on the floor, or lie down if you prefer. Focus in on the words in the script. Keeping your eyes closed may be helpful. When you've reached the end of the visualization, take a few more cleansing breaths before opening your eyes.

The Mountain

You're sitting on top of a mountain, at a place where you can see for miles all around you. The air is fresh and cool. You take a deep breath and enjoy the smell of the forest down below and all around you. You are wearing comfortable pants, a light sweater, socks, and shoes. You feel energized and light. The forest below you seems as though it is endless, like it goes on forever. It is autumn, and the leaves on the trees are many beautiful colors. You see red, orange, yellow, and green leaves. You can feel the dirt on your hands, which are resting beside you, touching the ground beneath you. The dirt is soft and smooth. You can hear birds singing. The sky is very blue, with no clouds in sight. In the distance, you can hear a waterfall. You take in a deep breath and smell the wonderful pine trees that are growing at the top of the mountain. The smell is refreshing and soothing. You close your eyes and take a few more breaths. You feel very calm and peaceful.

The Park

It's early in the morning on a beautiful spring day. You have arrived at the park before there is much activity. You find a comfortable spot on the grass and sit down to enjoy the morning sun. Although it's warm out, you feel a nice, refreshing breeze passing through your hair. Your skin is soaking up the early morning sunshine, and you feel at peace. There are several large oak trees nearby, and you see squirrels running up and down them. You don't hear anything, except perhaps the breeze itself as it rustles the leaves on the trees. You smell the dew on the grass. It is no longer wet, but the dewy smell lingers, with its fresh, early morning scent. The sun is still rising. The colors are beautiful in the sky. There are a few small clouds. It looks like it will be a lovely day. You spread a blanket out on the grass and lie down, with just your bare feet touching the grass. You look up at the sky and see a flock of birds flying. You feel happy, calm, and completely relaxed.

The Lake

You're sitting on a small beach that overlooks a beautiful lake. It is tranquil on the lake, with little ripples occasionally showing where the fish are swimming. You feel the sand beneath your body, with your feet digging into the soft, warm grains of sand. You feel the sand between your toes. The sand is practically white. Its smoothness calms your senses. You look out onto the lake and see a sailboat. It's sailing peacefully in the summer breeze. The day is warm and the sun feels good. You stand up and walk toward the lake. You slowly step into the lake, allowing the water to reach just above your ankles. It's cool and refreshing. As you walk a bit deeper into the water, your knees and hips are now wet. You love the calmness of the water. There are no waves, just clear, blue water. It is the perfect temperature on this warm summer day. You take a deep breath and fill your lungs with the fresh air. You feel totally relaxed and alive.

Muscle Relaxation

Now let's move on to exercises that help relax your muscles. Progressive muscle relaxation involves tightening and releasing, or tensing and relaxing, various muscles in your body. This technique was developed by Dr. Edmund Jacobson in the early 1920s based on his belief that, because anxiety and muscular tension often go hand in hand, we can decrease anxiety by learning how to relax our muscles. Dr. Joseph Wolpe, one of the founders of behavior therapy, took Jacobson's idea a step further (Poppen 1998) and developed a method for treating certain types of anxiety. Called *systematic desensitization*, this technique involves imaginary or real exposure to a feared stimulus while simultaneously relaxing the muscles. Dr. Wolpe found that anxiety was incompatible with a fully relaxed state, explaining why this technique is useful for helping people overcome fears, phobias, and anxiety.

Progressive Muscle Relaxation

Before beginning progressive muscle relaxation, be sure you're wearing comfortable, loose-fitting clothing. Find a quiet place where you can get comfortable. This may be inside your house, or even outside in a quiet spot in your backyard or the park. It's important to minimize distractions, so be sure to turn off your computer, cell phone, pager, radio, television, or anything else that may disturb you.

Next, sit or lie down in a comfortable position in which your entire body is supported. For a seated position, sitting in a recliner or on a sofa propped up with pillows works well. If you'd like to lie down, try your bed, the sofa, the floor, or even a blanket on the grass. Just remember that, like the other relaxation exercises you've learned so far, progressive muscle relaxation is meant to help you relax, *not* make you fall asleep.

During this exercise, you'll tighten and then release sixteen different groups of muscles. Each time you tighten, or tense, a muscle group, try to do so for ten seconds. Each time you release, or relax, a muscle group, try to do so for fifteen seconds. If you feel pain in any muscles as you're tensing them, decrease the level of tension slightly until you're more comfortable. If you continue to have pain there, skip that muscle group. If you have an injury, such as a pulled muscle, or any other medical condition that might make it inadvisable to tense your muscles, consult with your doctor before you try this exercise.

Take a few deep breaths before beginning this exercise. Although you can progress through your muscles in a different order if you prefer, this exercise will start with your toes and gradually work up to your head and face:

1. **Toes.** Curl your toes, digging them into the floor. Try not to tense your legs while you do this. Hold your toes in this position for ten seconds, counting to ten slowly. Then release your toes upward and relax. Count slowly to fifteen, keeping your toes relaxed.

2. **Feet and calves.** Point your toes and hold for ten seconds. Relax your feet for fifteen seconds.

3. **Shins.** Contract your shin muscles by flexing your feet upward. Do this slowly so you don't get a cramp. Keep your feet flexed upward for ten seconds, and then release for fifteen seconds.

4. **Thighs.** Contract your thigh muscles as tightly as you can by either extending your legs forward and raising them while tensing them, or simply by squeezing the muscles in your thighs tightly. Hold for ten seconds, and then relax for fifteen seconds.

5. **Buttocks.** Tense and squeeze your buttock muscles for ten seconds. Relax for fifteen seconds and feel the tension being released.

6. **Stomach.** Tighten your abdominal muscles by pulling in your stomach as much as you can for ten seconds. Keep tensing the muscles as you count. Relax and release for fifteen seconds, allowing your stomach muscles to fully relax.

7. **Back.** Arch your back while still keeping your shoulders supported. Hold for ten seconds, and then release for fifteen seconds. If you have a back injury or if this causes pain, skip this one.

8. **Chest.** Take a long, deep breath, tighten your chest muscles, and hold for ten seconds. Exhale and relax for fifteen seconds, breathing comfortably and normally for a few more breaths.

9. **Hands.** Squeeze your hands into fists for ten seconds, then allow your fingers to relax and extend for fifteen seconds.

10. **Biceps and triceps.** Tense your biceps by bringing your forearms up, like when you're "showing your muscles." Hold for ten seconds, and then release, allowing your hands to drop down to your sides and relax for fifteen seconds. Next, tighten your triceps muscles by straightening your arms out, contracting the backs of your upper arms, and holding for ten seconds. Then release for fifteen seconds.

11. **Shoulders.** Tighten and squeeze your shoulders back, holding for ten seconds. Then allow your shoulders to slump forward, relaxing, for fifteen seconds. If this causes pain or if you have a shoulder injury, you can skip this one.

12. **Neck.** Straighten your shoulders and keep them relaxed while turning your head slowly to the right side. Turn your head as far as you can and then hold it there for ten seconds. Bring your head back to a neutral position and relax for fifteen seconds. Repeat on the left side, turning your head as far as you can and holding it there for ten seconds. Release and let your head face forward for fifteen seconds. Next, drop your chin into your chest and hold it there for ten seconds. Then relax your neck muscles for fifteen seconds.

13. **Mouth.** Open your jaw as much as you can, stretching your mouth open wide. Hold for ten seconds, and then relax, closing your mouth for fifteen seconds. Next, smile as widely as you can, stretching your lips to the sides, and hold for ten seconds. Release and relax for fifteen seconds.

14. **Tongue.** Touch your tongue to the roof of your mouth and dig it in for ten seconds, then relax for fifteen seconds. Next, dig your tongue into the bottom of your mouth for ten seconds, and then relax for fifteen seconds.

15. **Eyes.** Open your eyes as wide as you can and hold for ten seconds, then relax for fifteen seconds. Next, shut your eyes tightly and hold for ten seconds, then keep your eyes closed, but relax them for fifteen seconds.

16. **Forehead.** Raise your eyebrows as high as you can, tightening the muscles in your forehead. Hold for ten seconds, and then release for fifteen seconds, bringing your eyebrows back down and smoothing out your forehead.

Try practicing progressive muscle relaxation every day for at least one week. Many people benefit by practicing this exercise at least twice daily. Once you're familiar with the exercise, you can pick and choose which muscles to tense and relax and tailor it to your individual needs.

Relaxing Your Muscles, Calming Your Thoughts, and Focusing On Your Breathing

Now that you've learned diaphragmatic breathing, deep breathing, guided imagery, and progressive muscle relaxation, you can combine these techniques into a relaxation exercise that will help you relax your muscles, calm your thoughts, and focus on slow, comfortable breathing. You may find it helpful to record this exercise so that you can practice it easily while listening, rather than having to read through the exercise or remember the process. Where a pause is indicated, pause for about five seconds. Begin by getting into a comfortable position in which your body is fully supported and closing your eyes.

Muscle, Thought, and Breath Relaxation Exercise

You are resting with your eyes closed. All of the parts of your body are supported, so there's no need to tense any muscle. Relax as much as you can (pause).

Focus your attention on your right hand and release whatever tension you may have there (pause). Relax all of your other muscles as much as you can (pause). Relax the muscles in your right forearm, feeling more and more relaxed (pause). Breathe slowly and calmly, relaxing more and more (pause).

Release the tension in your arm muscles, more and more deeply. Relax (pause). Now relax the muscles in your right upper arm Relax them as much as you can. Continue relaxing your entire right arm, your right hand, and your fingers. Relax as much as you can (pause). Relax. While continuing to relax your right arm and hand, focus your attention on your left hand. Relax your left hand as much as you can (pause). Feel the relaxation in your left arm as your muscles are beginning to relax, more and more deeply (pause). Release the tension, more and more profoundly. Relax more and more (pause). Continue to relax more and more, much more (pause). Breathe slowly and deeply, relaxing more and more (pause).

Now relax both of your shoulders and feel the weight lift. Feel the relaxation inside your shoulders, arms, hands, and fingers, calming you more and more (pause). Release the weight from your muscles, more and more (pause). You feel warmth in your muscles as you relax them more and more deeply. Your breathing is slow and even.

Now move to the muscles of your face. Smooth out your forehead. Relax those muscles more and more (pause). As you think of relaxing those muscles, you feel relaxation spreading through them slowly and gradually. Your eyes remain lightly closed (pause). The relaxation is slowly moving to your cheeks, releasing all tension (pause). Your jaw and tongue are relaxed, more and more deeply (pause). Relax as much as you can. With each breath, you release more and more tension. With each breath, you relax more and more (pause). Feel the relaxation moving to your neck, then down to your chest, while you continue relaxing more and more (pause). When you feel that you can release even more tension, simply relax as much as you can, more and more deeply (pause).

Your breathing is calm, slow, and regular, releasing more and more tension each time you exhale (pause). Your chest is relaxed. Relax down to your stomach, feeling more and more relaxed (pause). Relax as much as you can. Relax. Feel the relaxation in your hips, lower back, and buttocks while still resting comfortably. Relax more and more deeply (pause). The relaxation is now moving to your thighs and legs. You feel more and more relaxed (pause). More and more relaxed. More deeply relaxed. You are continuing to relax more deeply, more and more (pause). More and more. With each breath, you continue to relax more and more, releasing all of the tension inside your body (pause). Now relax your lower legs and your feet, relaxing more and more (pause). To help you relax a bit more, I will count backward from 10 to 1. When I say each number, see if you can relax more and more each time. Even when you think it's impossible to relax further, continue to try to relax more and more, enjoying more calm and relaxation (pause).

10, relax your body more and more (pause).

9, more and more deeply relaxed (pause).

8, slow and deep breathing, more and more relaxed (pause).

7, more and more (pause).

6, relax your whole body, feeling more and more relaxed (pause).

5, relaxing more and more deeply, breathing slowly and deeply, relaxing your entire body (pause).

4, all of your body feeling more and more relaxed, feeling warm and alive, feeling more and more calm (pause).

3, relaxing more and more deeply, calmness all around you, feeling more and more relaxed (pause).

2, more and more deeply relaxed, taking slow, deep breaths (pause).

1, continue relaxing your body like this, more and more (pause).

Now I want you to think of the word "peace" every time you breathe. I want you to relax every time you breathe and repeat the word "peace" in your head. That way, you will associate the word "peace" in your head with the peaceful state you are now in. Every time you breathe, I want you to think in silence the word "peace." Do this in your head until I speak to you again (pause for three minutes).

Very good. This exercise is now finished. I am going to count from 10 to 1, and when I arrive at the number 1, you will open your eyes and feel calm, relaxed, and awake. 10...9...8...7...6...5...4...3...2...1... Open your eyes; you are awake.

PRACTICE MAKES PERFECT

In order to really learn the relaxation techniques in this section, you need to practice them often. They can help you to cope with stress and will promote a healthier lifestyle. If you want these exercises to work for you when you're feeling anxious or stressed, you need to practice them at other times first. Don't feel frustrated if you have difficulty learning these techniques at first, and don't give up too quickly. It may take a dozen times of practicing the breathing exercises, for example, before you can consistently do them correctly and actually feel more relaxed.

It's also okay to alter the exercises to meet your needs. For example, if you want to replace the word "peace" in the last exercise with the word "calm" because you associate your state of mind during that exercise with calmness, then you should do it. These exercises need not be adhered to so strictly. Instead, you should adjust them so that they make sense and work for you. The instructions provided simply offer general guidelines. Explore these and various other relaxation techniques to find what's best for you, then start incorporating those exercises into your life as needed.

Making Time to Relax

Do you think the exercises in this chapter would be useful to you, but think you can't find the time to do them on a regular basis? Do you think setting aside time for relaxation exercises will be just one more thing to add to your to-do list? If so, fill out the following questionnaire to figure out how you might be able to squeeze in some time to relax each day.

How many hours of television do you watch each day?

_____

How much time do you spend talking on the telephone daily?

_____

How much time each day do you spend on the computer doing nonwork activities like checking e-mail or surfing the Internet?

_____

What other daily activities do you do that consume a lot of your time and energy? Are all of them necessary on a daily basis, or can you limit some of them to weekends or other specific times?

_____

_____

_____

Now look carefully at your answers to these questions. Do you spend too much time talking on the telephone? Do you turn on the television to watch a favorite program and then spend hours watching other shows as well? Do you sometimes turn on the television simply because you're bored and can't think of other things to do? Do you spend a lot of time on the computer? If so, cut back on some of these activities to free up time for relaxation exercises.

After talking with his doctor about how stressed-out he felt, Derrick decided to make some changes in his life. He started going to work a bit earlier each morning so that he could be home in time to help his wife at dinnertime. While she started cooking, Derrick took the kids to the playground so they could spend some time together and enjoy the fresh air. Derrick also realized that his weight was a problem, so he decided to join a group of friends who played basketball every Saturday morning. He also found that he could relax each day over lunch by walking to a nearby park and eating outside, rather than working at his desk while eating, as he'd done for years. Derrick realized that watching TV for several hours each night wasn't very productive, and also wasn't contributing to his well-being, so he started doing relaxation exercises in the evening hours after the kids went to bed. His wife saw the difference this made in Derrick and started joining him in his nightly relaxation sessions. Their relationship actually became stronger as a result of doing this, and they decided that once a month they'd hire a babysitter and have a "date night" for just the two of them. By learning the importance of relaxation and balance in his life, Derrick started to feel better both physically and mentally and eventually realized that he wasn't obsessing about his problems and stress while lying in bed at night. He was heading in the right direction and starting to get better sleep.

SUMMING UP

We all need balance in our lives. Learning to incorporate relaxing activities and relaxation exercises into your schedule on a daily basis will benefit your mind and your body. It's up to you to take the next step and begin practicing what you've learned in this chapter. If you think you don't have enough time to relax each day, you're not alone; many people feel this way. But if you make it a priority, you can surely find fifteen or twenty minutes a day to do a relaxation exercise. As you start to experience the benefits of relaxation, you may enjoy it so much that you create even more time in your daily life to relax. You don't have to make drastic changes in your life, but you should give yourself the time and relaxation you need.

CHAPTER 6

Sleep Logs

As part of this sleep program, it's important to keep track of your sleep-wake patterns in a systematic, routine way. For that reason, you'll be keeping a sleep log—a diary in which you record your sleep habits, sleep patterns, and overall sleep time. You'll keep track of the number of hours you sleep each night, when you turn out the lights, fall asleep, and get up out of bed to start your day, and any awakenings you may have. A sleep log is essential for helping you keep track of good nights versus bad nights, which will allow you to figure out what kinds of factors may contribute to a poor night of sleep for you. For example, some people have found that when they talk on the phone late in the evening, their sleep is more likely to be disrupted. This could be due to getting excited about the conversation, talking about issues that aren't relaxing or conducive to sleep, or even just lying in bed thinking about the conversation. Other people find that when they have a few glasses of wine in the late evening, their sleep may be more disrupted compared to nights when they don't drink more than one glass of wine.

By helping you become more aware of what factors contribute to a good night of sleep versus a bad one, the log will allow you to make behavioral changes to promote better sleep. It will also give you an idea of how much sleep you average on a nightly basis. Don't just gloss over this chapter. A sleep log is an integral part of this program, and you'll need the information you record in your sleep log in order to implement the sleep restriction program in chapter 7.

WHEN AND HOW TO RECORD YOUR SLEEP

The best time to record your sleep is first thing in the morning after you get out of bed. Although you may be tempted to write in your sleep log if you wake up in the middle of the night, please don't do that. Taking notes in the middle of the night will only further disrupt your sleep, which would be counterproductive. Also, don't worry about being 100 percent accurate; I don't want you to be looking at the clock during the night. Again, that would be counterproductive, since looking at the clock only causes you to worry more about your sleep and sends an anxiety-provoking signal to your brain, which you want to avoid. Instead, just jot down what you remember about the previous night of sleep when you get up in the morning. Although this won't provide an absolutely perfect record of your sleep, it's good enough for our purposes. The point of the sleep log is ultimately to help you sleep better, so filling it out shouldn't involve doing anything that could make your sleep worse!

While the purpose of different sleep logs is the same—to gather and document information about your sleep-wake patterns—various formats are available. Some sleep logs are more quantitative in nature, focusing mostly on the actual number of hours you sleep each night. Others are more qualitative, with space for recording details about different factors affecting your sleep. I've included two different formats, along with an example of each, so you can choose the format you prefer. The first is a more visual or graphic format that allows you to see the bigger picture of your sleep, and the second is more detailed, asking specific questions about your sleep and daytime activities to help increase your awareness of the factors affecting your sleep. I've put the filled-out examples first, to help you see how to use each log. Both examples record the same information so you can compare the two ways of keeping a sleep log.

Sample of Visual Sleep Log

Record the date on the left-hand side of each row. Since the sleep log crosses over two days, indicate the date of the day when you record the information—the day after your night of sleep. Use a down arrow (⇩) to indicate when you turn out the lights each night, or when you go back to bed after a nighttime awakening. Shade in when you actually sleep, whether for a full hour or parts of an hour. Use an up arrow (⇧) to indicate when you wake up in the morning, and also any time that you wake up during the night. You should also indicate if you take any naps by shading those spaces. Use the following codes to indicate other factors that may be affecting your sleep:

C = Caffeine   N = Nicotine

E = Exercise   M = Sleep medications

F = Food   A = Alcohol

R = Relaxation exercises   O = Out of bed during the night

S = Stressful event (at work, home, or anywhere else)

Here's an example of how to use this sleep log. The first date is marked as 5/20-5/21. The information is for the night of 5/20, continuing into the day of 5/21. The person exercised (E) from 6 to 7 p.m. She ate dinner (F) and drank alcohol (A) at 8 p.m. She took a sleeping medication (M) at around 9 p.m and turned out the lights (⇩) at 10:30 p.m.. She fell asleep by 11 p.m. but woke up at 2 a.m. and got out of bed (⇧ and O). At 3:30 a.m., she went back to bed (⇩) and fell asleep by 4 a.m. She then slept from 4 to 7 a.m. (⇧). She ate breakfast at 8 a.m. Later the same day, she took a nap after lunch (F), from 1 to 2 p.m. On the next line is 5/21 continuing into 5/22. She exercised from 6 to 7 p.m. and ate dinner (F) and drank alcohol (A) at 7 p.m. She took a sleeping medication at 9 p.m. and got into bed at 11:30 p.m. She fell asleep by 12 midnight and slept until 4 a.m. She remained in her bed, awake, until 6 a.m., when she fell asleep until 7 a.m. She ate breakfast (F) and had coffee (C) at 8 a.m. She experienced stress (S) at work at 10 a.m., ate lunch (F) at 12 noon, had an espresso at 2 p.m. (C), and had another stressful (S) event at work at 3 p.m. Her total hours of sleep are recorded at the end of each line.

Date	6 pm	7 pm	8 pm	9 pm	10 pm	11 pm	12 am	1 am	2 am	3 am	4 am	5 am	6 am	7 am	8 am	9 am	10 am	11 am	12 pm	1 pm	2 pm	3 pm	4 pm	5 pm	Total
5/20-5/21	E		F/A	M	⇨				⇧O	⇨				⇦	F				F⇩		⇦				7
5/21-5/22	E	F/A	A	M		⇨					⇦	⇨		⇦	F/C		S		F		C	S			5
5/22-5/23	A	F/A	A		M	⇨				⇦	⇨	⇧⇨				⇧F				F			E		5
5/23-5/24		F	R		⇨					⇧⇨				⇦	F				F						7
5/24-5/25	S	F	F	R	⇨			⇧O		⇨				⇦	F/C			S	F					E	5
5/25-5/26	E	F			⇨						⇦	O		F/C					F						4
5/26-5/27	E	F	R			⇨							⇦	F/C				F							6
Average																									5.6

91

Visual Sleep Log

Record the date on the left-hand side of each row. Since the sleep log crosses over two days, indicate the date of the day when you record the information—the day after your night of sleep. Use a down arrow (⇩) to indicate when you turn out the lights each night, or when you go back to bed after a nighttime awakening. Shade in when you actually sleep, whether for a full hour or parts of an hour. Use an up arrow (⇧) to indicate when you wake up in the morning, and also any time that you wake up during the night. You should also indicate if you take any naps by shading those spaces. Use the following codes to indicate other factors that may be affecting your sleep:

C = Caffeine   N = Nicotine

E = Exercise   M = Sleep medications

F = Food   A = Alcohol

R = Relaxation exercises   O = Out of bed during the night

S = Stressful event (at work, home, or anywhere else)

Date	6 pm	7 pm	8 pm	9 pm	10 pm	11 pm	12 am	1 am	2 am	3 am	4 am	5 am	6 am	7 am	8 am	9 am	10 am	11 am	12 pm	1 pm	2 pm	3 pm	4 pm	5 pm	Total
Average																									

Sample of Descriptive Sleep Log

Fill out this sleep log daily, answering each of the questions as best you can. You can answer the questions about your day anytime during the day, but answer the questions about your night as soon as possible after you wake up and get out of bed in the morning. For example, for the question on stress, record any stressful events that occurred during the day before your night of sleep.

Here's an example of how to use this version of the sleep log, using the same information recorded in the previous example.

Date	5/21	5/22	5/23	5/24	5/25	5/26	5/27
Day of the week	Thursday	Friday	Saturday	Sunday	Monday	Tuesday	Wednesday
Questions about your day							
Did anything stressful happen during your day (at home, at work, or elsewhere)? If yes, describe what happened.	yes □ no ☒	yes ☒ no □ — At 10 a.m., stress with client at work; at 3 p.m., fight with coworker.	yes □ no ☒	yes □ no ☒	yes ☒ no □ — At 11:30 a.m., I heard some bad news from a friend.	yes □ no ☒	yes □ no ☒
Did you nap? If so, for how long and at what time?	yes ☒ no □ — 1 hour 1-2 p.m.	yes □ no ☒	yes □ no ☒	yes □ no ☒	yes □ no ☒	yes □ no ☒	yes □ no ☒
Did you do any relaxation exercises? If yes, at what time?	yes □ no ☒	yes □ no ☒	yes □ no ☒	yes ☒ no □ — 8 p.m.	yes ☒ no □ — 8 p.m.	yes □ no ☒	yes ☒ no □ — 8 p.m.
Did you have any caffeine after 12 noon? If yes, at what time?	yes □ no ☒	yes ☒ no □ — 2:30 p.m.	yes □ no ☒	yes □ no ☒	yes □ no ☒	yes □ no ☒	yes □ no ☒
Did you exercise? If yes, at what time?	yes ☒ no □ — 6-7 p.m.	yes ☒ no □ — 6-7 p.m.	yes ☒ no □ — 4:30-5 p.m.	yes □ no ☒	yes ☒ no □ — 5-6 p.m.	yes □ no ☒	yes ☒ no □ — 6-7 p.m.
Did you have any alcohol? If yes, at what time?	yes ☒ no □ — 8 p.m.	yes ☒ no □ — 7 p.m.	yes ☒ no □ — 6:30 p.m., 7 & 8 p.m.	yes □ no ☒	yes □ no ☒	yes □ no ☒	yes □ no ☒
Did you use any nicotine after 5 p.m.? If yes, how much?	yes □ no ☒	yes □ no ☒	yes □ no ☒	yes □ no ☒	yes □ no ☒	yes □ no ☒	yes □ no ☒
Did you feel sleepy during the day?	yes ☒ no □	yes ☒ no □	yes ☒ no □	yes □ no ☒	yes ☒ no □	yes ☒ no □	yes □ no ☒

Rate and describe your mood 1=poor, 2=fair, 3=good, 4=excellent	3 – good day	1 – lots of stress at work	2 – bad night's sleep and still stressed from work	4 – great with lots of energy	3 – feeling pretty good, although had some upsetting news from a friend	2	3 – trying to relax more
How was your overall functioning during the day? (1=poor, 2=fair, 3=good, 4=excellent)	2—too sleepy	2	2	4	3	3	4
Questions about your night							
Did you take any sleeping medication? Specify which drug, what dose, and when you took it.	yes ☑ no □ Ambien 10 mg 9 p.m.	yes ☑ no □ Ambien 10 mg 9 p.m.	yes ☑ no □ Ambien 10 mg 10:15 p.m.	yes □ no ☑	yes ☑ no □ Ambien 10 mg 9 p.m.	yes ☑ no □	yes □ no ☑
What time did you turn off the lights?	10:30 p.m.	11:30 p.m.	11:30 p.m.	10:30 p.m.	10:20 p.m.	10:30 p.m.	11:30 p.m.
How long did it take you to fall asleep?	30 min.	30 min.	90 min.	30 min.	30 min.	90 min.	30 min.
How many times did you wake up during the night? For how long?	1 time 2 hours	1 time 2 hours	1 time 3 hours	1 time 1 hour	1 time 3 hours	1 time I didn't go back to sleep.	0
What time did you get up out of bed in the morning to start your day?	7 a.m.	7 a.m.	9:15 a.m.	7 a.m.	7:10 a.m.	4 a.m.	6 a.m.
How many hours total did you sleep at night?	6 hours	5 hours	5 hours	7 hours	5 hours	4 hours	6 hours
What was the quality of your sleep? (1=poor, 2=fair, 3=good, 4=very good, 5=excellent)	2	2	1	4	2	1	5
Estimated total sleep time (Nighttime sleep plus daytime naps)	6+1=7	5	5	7	5	4	6

Descriptive Sleep Log

Fill out sleep log daily, answering each of the questions as best you can. You can answer the questions about your day anytime during the day, but answer the questions about your night as soon as possible after you wake up and get out of bed in the morning. For example, for the question on stress, record any stressful events that occurred during the day before your night of sleep.

Date							
Day of the week							
Questions about your day							
Did anything stressful happen during your day (at home, at work, or elsewhere)? If yes, describe what happened.	yes ☐ no ☐	yes ☐ no ☐	yes ☐ no ☐	yes ☐ no ☐	yes ☐ no ☐	yes ☐ no ☐	yes ☐ no ☐
Did you nap? If so, for how long and at what time?	yes ☐ no ☐	yes ☐ no ☐	yes ☐ no ☐	yes ☐ no ☐	yes ☐ no ☐	yes ☐ no ☐	yes ☐ no ☐
Did you do any relaxation exercises? If yes, at what time?	yes ☐ no ☐	yes ☐ no ☐	yes ☐ no ☐	yes ☐ no ☐	yes ☐ no ☐	yes ☐ no ☐	yes ☐ no ☐
Did you have any caffeine after 12 noon? If yes, at what time?	yes ☐ no ☐	yes ☐ no ☐	yes ☐ no ☐	yes ☐ no ☐	yes ☐ no ☐	yes ☐ no ☐	yes ☐ no ☐
Did you exercise? If yes, at what time?	yes ☐ no ☐	yes ☐ no ☐	yes ☐ no ☐	yes ☐ no ☐	yes ☐ no ☐	yes ☐ no ☐	yes ☐ no ☐
Did you have any alcohol? If yes, at what time?	yes ☐ no ☐	yes ☐ no ☐	yes ☐ no ☐	yes ☐ no ☐	yes ☐ no ☐	yes ☐ no ☐	yes ☐ no ☐
Did you use any nicotine after 5 p.m.? If yes, how much?	yes ☐ no ☐	yes ☐ no ☐	yes ☐ no ☐	yes ☐ no ☐	yes ☐ no ☐	yes ☐ no ☐	yes ☐ no ☐
Did you feel sleepy during the day?	yes ☐ no ☐	yes ☐ no ☐	yes ☐ no ☐	yes ☐ no ☐	yes ☐ no ☐	yes ☐ no ☐	yes ☐ no ☐
Rate and describe your mood 1=poor, 2=fair, 3=good, 4=excellent							

How was your overall functioning during the day? (1=poor, 2=fair, 3=good, 4=excellent)							
Questions about your night							
Did you take any sleeping medication? Specify which drug, what dose, and when you took it.	yes ☐ no ☐	yes ☐ no ☐	yes ☐ no ☐	yes ☐ no ☐	yes ☐ no ☐	yes ☐ no ☐	yes ☐ no ☐
What time did you turn off the lights?							
How long did it take you to fall asleep?							
How many times did you wake up during the night? For how long?							
What time did you get up out of bed in the morning to start your day?							
How many hours total did you sleep at night?							
What was the quality of your sleep? (1=poor, 2=fair, 3=good, 4=very good, 5=excellent)							
Estimated total sleep time (night-time sleep plus daytime naps)							

KEEPING YOUR SLEEP LOG

Since there is only space for seven days on each of the sleep logs, you need to make copies so that you can continue to use them for longer than just one week. If you prefer to come up with your own format, that's fine as long as you include space to record, at a minimum, the time when you turned the lights out, approximate time you feel asleep, when you woke up and got out of bed to start your day, time and length of any awakenings during the night, duration of any naps, and total sleep time. After you've decided which sleep log you prefer, keep track of your sleep every day for an entire week before you begin to evaluate your log. You need to gather enough baseline information before you start making too many changes. After you've kept your sleep log for one week, you can move on to the next section, on evaluating it.

ANALYZING YOUR SLEEP LOG

Now that you've completed your sleep log for one week, you can begin to examine what patterns occur and the factors that may be contributing to your poor sleep. Do you see anything in particular that affected your sleep-wake cycle, or any factors that led to good nights versus bad nights?

Figuring Out What's Affecting Your Sleep

Let's go through the following exercise to help you become more aware of what factors may be affecting your sleep.

What effect did stress have on your sleep? Did it cause you to have trouble falling asleep or staying asleep?

_____

_____

Did you try any relaxation exercises? If so, did they impact your sleep?

_____

_____

Did you exercise during the week? If so, did you notice a difference in your sleep depending on whether you exercised and the time of day you exercised (for example, morning versus afternoon or evening)?

_____

_____

Did you consume anything with caffeine after noon? If so, what was your sleep pattern like? Any trouble falling asleep or staying asleep?

_____

_____

Did you drink alcohol during the week? If so, how did it impact your sleep? For example, did you find it easier to fall asleep but then have more awakenings during the night or more restless sleep?

_____

_____

Did the time that you ate dinner affect your sleep (late versus early)? Did the type of meal affect your sleep (light versus heavy)?

_____

_____

Did you take any sleeping pills? If so, did they improve your sleep? After taking sleeping medications, how quickly did you fall asleep and how long did you sleep? Did you awaken during the night?

_____

_____

Did you take any naps during the day? If so, how did that affect your nighttime sleep? Was it more difficult for you to fall asleep or stay asleep at night after taking a nap in the day?

_____

_____

Did you go to bed at the same time every night? If not, did your bedtime fluctuate by more than an hour from night to night?

_____

_____

Did you wake up at the same time every day? If not, did your rise time vary by more than an hour from day to day?

_____

_____

Did you sleep any better or worse on weekends versus weekdays?

Now that you've examined some of the factors likely to be affecting your sleep, it's time to make a few behavioral changes. All of these questions, and your answers to them, are intended to help you realize where you can make changes that will improve your sleep. If you had a stressful day, did you try doing any relaxation exercises in the evening hours? If you noticed that exercising at 8 p.m. made it difficult for you to fall asleep, then you should change your exercise time to either earlier in the evening (ideally at least four hours before bedtime) or in the morning. Similarly, if you discover that the caffeinated beverage you drank with dinner disrupted your sleep, it's time to reduce or eliminate all caffeine within twelve hours of bedtime. What about alcohol? Did you notice that one glass of wine was fine, but when you had several glasses you had more disrupted sleep? Meals can affect your sleep as well, particularly dinner. Did you notice any links between what you ate or when you ate it and your sleep the following night? And what about sleep medications? If you're taking them, it's worthwhile to analyze how much they're actually helping you, given the many potential downsides to these medications.

Did napping affect your sleep at night? Remember that you only need a certain amount of sleep in a twenty-four-hour period, so taking a snooze during the day can make it harder to sleep at night. Did your sleep schedule change from night to night? If so, that could be another reason for your poor sleep. For example, allowing yourself to sleep late on the weekends can make it difficult for you to fall asleep the next night. Did you find that you slept better on the weekends, when you didn't have as much to worry about or do? If so, adding some relaxation exercises to your daily schedule and creating a calming bedtime routine may help you.

Calculating Your Total Sleep Time and Sleep Efficiency

There are two main reasons for keeping a sleep log. The first is to figure out why you have trouble sleeping by examining the many different factors that may be affecting your sleep, which we've just done in the previous exercise. The second reason for keeping a sleep log is to calculate your total sleep time and your sleep efficiency. *Total sleep time* is exactly what it sounds like: the amount of time you spend sleeping in your bed at night, plus any naps you may take during the day. *Sleep efficiency* refers to the percentage of time you spend actually sleeping in your bed at night versus the total amount of time you spend in your bed. For example, if you sleep 85 percent of the time you're in bed at night, your sleep efficiency is 85 percent; the other 15 percent of the time you're awake in bed. Ideally, your sleep efficiency should be above 90 percent.

Most people with insomnia have poor sleep efficiency, meaning they spend too much time lying in bed when they aren't sleeping. As discussed in previous chapters, spending too much time in bed while you're awake is part of the reason that your mind and body now associate your bed with being awake rather than being asleep. The first step in changing this conditioned association is to calculate your average total sleep time and your sleep efficiency. Here's how to do it: Assuming that you're doing your calculations based on an entire week's worth of data in your sleep log, first add up the total number of hours you slept during the week. Then add up the total number of hours you spent in bed during the week, including any time when you were lying in bed but not sleeping. Then simply divide your total sleep time by your total number of hours in bed. If you haven't done so already, go ahead and actually calculate your sleep efficiency based on a week's worth of data in your sleep log:

Total sleep time for the week (TST): _____

Total time in bed for the week (TIB): _____

Sleep efficiency (SE); TST divided by TIB: _____

The preceding method is used in chapter 7. However, you can also calculate your average total sleep time by dividing your total sleep time by the number of days for which you recorded your sleep. Then do the same with your total number of hours in bed. Finally, divide your average total sleep time by your average number of hours in bed to come up with your average sleep efficiency. Either way, you'll come up with the same number for your efficiency. So, if you averaged six hours of sleep each night, but you spent an average of eight hours in bed each night, your sleep efficiency is 6 divided by 8, which is .75, or 75 percent. That means you spent 75 percent of your time in bed actually sleeping and the other 25 percent awake.

SUMMING UP

Keeping track of your sleep with a sleep log is an important part of the program in this book. Doing so will help you pinpoint factors that contribute to a good night of sleep versus a bad night for you. You can then use this information to make the appropriate changes. In addition, a sleep log will provide information you can use to calculate your sleep efficiency and then record your progress in improving that efficiency. By using a sleep log, you're taking an active role in overcoming your insomnia and improving your overall sleep.

CHAPTER 7

Stimulus Control and Sleep Restriction

This chapter focuses on two important and complementary components of this sleep program: stimulus control and sleep restriction. Both involve making changes based on the information you've gathered in your sleep log. *Sleep restriction* involves restricting the amount of time you spend in bed to your average total sleep time. The goal of sleep restriction is to consolidate your sleep and improve your sleep efficiency so that you are actually sleeping most of the time you're in bed. This is combined with a behavioral approach called *stimulus control*, which is based on conditioning principles wherein a stimulus, such as your bed or bedroom, serves as a cue to reinforce subsequent behaviors, such as falling asleep or *not* falling asleep (Bootzin and Rider 2000). If you've spent many hours lying in your bed trying to fall asleep, or if you engage in stimulating activities in bed, such as reading, watching TV, eating, talking on the phone, or worrying, then you're actually reinforcing the conditioned response that when you get into your bed, you remain awake instead of falling asleep. In other words, by remaining in your bed for long periods of time when you aren't sleeping, you've created an association between your bed and *not* sleeping.

For good sleepers, stimuli such as the bed, bedtime, or the bedroom serve as cues that are associated with feeling sleepy and then going to sleep. For poor sleepers, however, the same stimuli are typically associated with arousal, frustration, and difficulty sleeping (Morin 1993). Stimulus control therapy for insomnia is intended to break these associations and create new, sleep-promoting associations.

STIMULUS CONTROL FOR INSOMNIA

Dr. Richard Bootzin started using stimulus control for insomnia in the 1970s. The idea behind this behavioral technique is twofold: First, you need to stop the current association between the cue or the setting (your bed or bedroom), the timing (bedtime), and the conditioned response (not falling asleep).

That means stopping behaviors that are incompatible with sleep, such as watching TV and reading in bed. Second, you need to replace that old association with a new one, where the bed or bedroom actually serves as a cue for you to fall asleep. Stimulus control works to undo the negative conditioned association that's making it harder for you to fall asleep and replace it with a positive association that makes it easier for you to fall asleep again.

Stimulus Control Instructions

Here are the basic guidelines for stimulus control for insomnia, incorporating the original instructions that Dr. Bootzin (1972) created:

1. Establish a nightly bedtime routine. Try to spend at least one hour before bedtime doing relaxing activities, such as quietly watching TV or reading a book (neither too exciting) in another room, or practicing deep breathing or other relaxation exercises. Limit stimulating activities such as talking on the telephone, working on the computer, vigorous physical activity, or doing any type of business-related work.

2. Only get into bed when you're actually feeling sleepy.

3. The bed is for sleep and sex only. Any other activities, such as reading, watching TV, talking on the phone, eating, using your laptop, and even worrying, aren't allowed in bed.

4. If you can't fall asleep in approximately fifteen to twenty minutes after lying in your bed, get up and go into another room. I say "approximately" because good sleep hygiene includes not looking at the clock. Don't worry about the exact number of minutes that you're lying in bed awake. You know your body pretty well, and if you feel wide awake, anxious, worried, or just like you've been tossing and turning for at least fifteen minutes, simply get up out of bed.

5. Find something boring to do, like reading a dull magazine article or book or watching an uninteresting television program. You can also do something relaxing, like listening to calming music or practicing relaxation exercises, including deep breathing, meditation, or guided imagery. Don't fall asleep on the couch or in a recliner. Don't do anything physically active during this time, because you don't want to jump-start your system into thinking it's time for you to start your day. Similarly, try to keep the lights off or very dim so you don't confuse your brain into thinking it's daytime.

6. When you feel sleepy again, go back to bed and give yourself a chance to fall asleep.

7. Repeat steps 4 through 6 as often as needed throughout the night.

8. Establish a wake-up time, set your alarm clock for that time every day, and get up when the alarm goes off, even if you slept poorly. Getting up at the same time every morning will help you establish a regular sleep-wake schedule.

9. Don't nap during the day.

Remember, the reason for stimulus control is to establish a better association between your bed and bedtime and a positive response: sleeping. The instructions above incorporate setting up a sleep-promoting environment and eliminating those activities in the bed that are lowering your chances of sleep. Although it can be difficult to force yourself out of bed when you are trying so hard to fall asleep, keep in mind that stimulus control works very well for those who do it. In fact, numerous studies report that stimulus control for insomnia is one of the most effective parts of insomnia treatment (Morin et al. 2006; Chesson et al. 1999; Morin, Hauri, et al. 1999). Be sure to continue keeping your sleep log on a daily basis while incorporating stimulus control.

Assessing Problems with Stimulus Control

Each morning when you get up out of bed, review the list below to see if you're following all of the stimulus control instructions for insomnia. You might even make a copy of this list and post it in a place where you'll see it every morning.

____ yes	____ no	1. Do you have a regular bedtime routine?
____ yes	____ no	2. Do you only go to bed when you actually feel sleepy?
____ yes	____ no	3. Are you watching TV, reading, worrying, or doing other activities in bed?
____ yes	____ no	4. Do you get up out of bed after fifteen to twenty minutes of not sleeping?
____ yes	____ no	5. After getting out of bed in the middle of the night, do you do something boring or relaxing?
____ yes	____ no	6. Do you only get back into bed when you feel sleepy?
____ yes	____ no	7. Do you get up at the same time every morning?
____ yes	____ no	8. Are you napping during the day?

Yes is the correct answer to all of these questions except for numbers 3 and 8. Let's briefly review why these are the correct answers.

For question 1, the correct answer is yes because establishing a relaxing, peaceful nighttime routine is an important way to set the stage for sleep by being relaxed and calm when you get into bed at night. By avoiding stimulating activities at bedtime and focusing on making the hour or so before bedtime more calm and relaxing, you'll be on your way to promoting a better night of sleep.

For question 2, the correct answer is yes, since you should only be getting into bed when you feel sleepy. As you're probably well aware by now, the more time you spend lying in bed trying to fall asleep, the more frustrated you'll become, and the more you'll associate your bed and bedtime with an anxiety and sleeplessness. By going to bed only when you feel sleepy, you increase your chances of falling asleep sooner.

For question 3, the correct answer is no, because your bed should be reserved for sleep and sex only. All other activities, such as reading, watching TV, eating, and worrying, should take place somewhere else. In order for your mind to associate your bed with a tranquil, quiet place that's conducive to sleep, you need to stop doing stimulating activities in bed.

For question 4, the correct answer is yes. Again, you don't want to spend much time lying in bed when you aren't actually sleeping so that you can change your association between sleeplessness and your bed, bedroom, or bedtime. If you lie awake in bed for too long, you'll become annoyed and frustrated. This isn't a good feeling to associate with your bed, so it's important to get out of bed and return only when you're feeling calm and sleepy.

For question 5, the correct answer is yes. It's important to try to engage in sleep-promoting behaviors if you get up in the middle of the night, which means doing something relaxing or boring. If you work on your computer, read an interesting book, watch a great movie, do laundry, or start cleaning your house, you aren't giving yourself a very good chance of feeling sleepy again.

For question 6, the correct answer is yes. Remember that you only want to get into bed when you're feeling sleepy. This rule is the same in the middle of the night as it is at the beginning of the night. Once you start yawning, notice your eyes becoming heavy, or feel like you could drift off to sleep, get back in bed.

For question 7, the correct answer is yes. By getting up at the same time each day, regardless of the number of hours of sleep you've had the night before, you'll build up a little bit of sleep debt. This will help you fall asleep more easily the next night. So even if you want to get up later one morning, try to be consistent and get up at the same time every day. This will increase your chances of better sleep.

For question 8, the correct answer is no. If you nap during the day, you'll undo the progress you're making on sleeping better at night. Remember, you only need a certain amount of sleep across a twenty-four-hour period and naps count as part of your total sleep time. If you nap during the day, you won't need as much sleep at night. So for now, try not to nap during the day.

SLEEP RESTRICTION FOR INSOMNIA

Now that you've learned about stimulus control, you're ready to start the next component of the sleep program: sleep restriction. As mentioned at the start of this chapter, sleep restriction involves limiting your time in bed to the total number of hours that you estimate you actually sleep each night, so you'll need to calculate your average total sleep time from your sleep log. You need to continue keeping your sleep log for the entire time that you're doing sleep restriction, as the information in the log is essential for devising the appropriate sleep restriction plan. The purpose of sleep restriction is to consolidate your sleep so that you go to sleep more quickly and awaken less often. This will allow you to have more restful, restorative sleep in the long run, but you should expect a minor amount of sleep loss at first (Spielman and Anderson 1999). Creating a small sleep debt is actually helpful, as it will make you feel sleepier at night. As a result, you should fall asleep more quickly and sleep more soundly.

Sleep restriction therapy was originally designed by Dr. Arthur Spielman as an answer to the problem most people with insomnia have: spending too much time in bed trying to fall asleep (Spielman, Saskin, and Thorpy 1987). Since poor sleepers remember from many previous bad nights that it usually takes them quite a while to fall asleep, they often get into bed earlier to give themselves enough time or extra time to sleep. In addition, they may lie awake in bed in the morning, hoping this will help them feel rested. But this extra time in bed just perpetuates the conditioned sleep problem.

As you can see, sleep restriction and stimulus control go hand-in-hand, which is why I've combined them in this chapter. Restricting the time you spend in bed each night to the average number of hours you actually sleep should improve your sleep efficiency so that sleep fills up more and more of the time you spend in bed. This reconditions your body to a regular sleep-wake schedule and helps you develop new and positive associations with your bed, bedtime, and sleep environment.

How to Implement Sleep Restriction

Let's take a look at Sleepless Susie for an example of how to do sleep restriction. First we'll use Susie's sleep log to calculate her total sleep time for each night and her average total sleep time, just like you'll need to do with your sleep log in order to start doing sleep restriction.

Sleepless Susie's Sleep Log

Date	6 pm	7 pm	8 pm	9 pm	10 pm	11 pm	12 am	1 am	2 am	3 am	4 am	5 am	6 am	7 am	8 am	9 am	10 am	11 am	12 pm	1 pm	2 pm	3 pm	4 pm	5 pm	Total
2/1						▓	▓	▓			▓	▓	▓							▓					
2/2							▓				▓	▓	▓												
2/3							▓	▓	▓	▓			▓	▓											
2/4		▓							▓	▓				▓											
2/5							▓	▓	▓			▓	▓												
2/6						▓	▓	▓				▓													
2/7						▓	▓	▓	▓	▓															
Average																									

During the week recorded here, Susie slept 7 hours, 4 hours, 6 hours, 5 hours, 5 hours, 4 hours, and 5 hours, respectively, for a total of 36 hours. To calculate Susie's average total sleep time, divide 36 by 7, since that's the number of days recorded on this sleep log. This gives the result 5.1 hours—Susie's average total sleep time across the week. To implement sleep restriction, Susie needs to restrict her time in bed to about 5 hours each night.

Susie chose to set her new bedtime as 12 midnight, with a rise time of 5 a.m. Since she didn't fall asleep before 12 midnight on four out of the seven nights, this seems like an appropriate bedtime for her. Restricting her sleep to only 5 hours each night means that even if she doesn't sleep for 5 hours straight, she's only allowed to be in bed from 12 midnight to 5 a.m. If she wakes up during this time and starts worrying about things, she should get out of bed after 15 minutes and do something boring or relaxing. In other words, the rules of stimulus control remain in place when you're doing sleep restriction.

Are You Worried About Doing Sleep Restriction?

If you're starting to feel nervous or apprehensive about sleep restriction, you're not alone. It can be scary to think that you're only allowed a restricted amount of time in bed each night, regardless of the number of hours you actually sleep—especially if you've been plagued by sleeplessness and sleep deprivation. Take heart in knowing that studies have shown sleep restriction to be an effective solution for insomnia (Morin et al. 2006; Spielman and Anderson 1999). Even if you get less sleep for a little while at the outset, soon your sleep will benefit. It can be tough to stick with it on the first few nights, before you start to experience the benefits, but soon you should start falling asleep more quickly, and your sleep should become more consolidated. Building up a bit of a sleep debt in the initial phase creates a stronger urge for you to fall asleep at bedtime, which is exactly what you want.

You need to be careful, however, not to let yourself fall asleep too early in the evening. If you feel very sleepy before your designated bedtime, try to stay active and busy until an hour or so before bedtime, when you can begin to unwind, relax, and prepare for bed. Definitely don't take any naps, because you don't want to undo the important work you're doing at night to improve your sleep. If you feel very sleepy during the day when you start your sleep restriction program, avoid any activities that could be dangerous, like driving or operating heavy machinery.

Sleep Restriction Guidelines for Week 1

Here are detailed instructions for the first week of your sleep restriction program:

1. Prior to starting sleep restriction, keep your sleep log for at least one week.

2. Calculate your total sleep time (TST) each night.

3. After at least one week, calculate your average total sleep time by adding up all of your nightly TSTs and dividing the grand total by the number of days.

4. Restrict your sleep to the average total sleep time you just calculated, but don't go below five hours. If your average TST falls below five hours, just use five as your average. And remember, your average TST is the maximum number of hours you're allowed to be in bed, regardless of how much of that time you spend sleeping.

5. Set your new bedtime and rise time using your average TST. For example, if your average TST is 6 hours, then you could go to bed at 11 p.m. and get up at 5 a.m., or go to bed at 12 midnight and get up at 6 a.m. Just pick the bedtime and rise time that fit your schedule best and that you are most likely to adhere to on a daily basis.

6. Follow the rules of stimulus control discussed earlier in this chapter. For example, if you're awake for more than 15 minutes in the middle of the night, get up and do something boring or relaxing. Similarly, don't read, watch TV, eat, talk on the phone, or worry in bed.

7. Even if you get up during the night, still restrict the amount of time you're allowed to be in bed to your average TST.

8. Set your alarm clock for the same time each day, and get up at that time.

9. No napping during the day!

10. Remember that sleep restriction involves restricting the amount of time you're allowed to be in bed each night. This is your "sleep window." But if you aren't sleepy during this time or find yourself tossing and turning, it's important that you get up out of bed and only go back to bed when you actually feel sleepy. You aren't required to stay in your bed during the entire "sleep window" each night, and in fact, it's counterproductive to do so if you don't feel sleepy.

11. Continue keeping your sleep log throughout your sleep restriction program.

Sleep Restriction Guidelines for After Week 1

You're probably wondering how long you'll need to implement sleep restriction and what to do after you're sleeping well for the number of hours you've restricted yourself to in bed. This depends on how quickly and efficiently your sleep restriction program works. The more you adhere to it while also following the stimulus control guidelines, the sooner you can expect to be sleeping better. Some people see positive changes in their sleep in as few as three or four nights, whereas it can take a couple of weeks for other people. Be patient and don't give up too early. These methods have been researched and proven to be very effective for insomnia, so you just need to give them a chance to start working on your body. Now let's take a closer look at how to adjust your sleep restriction program based on how well you sleep during week 1. Two different methods of implementing sleep restriction are provided so you can choose the one that suits you best: a method based on calculating your sleep efficiency and the "sleeping solidly" approach.

REVISING YOUR TIME IN BED BASED ON CALCULATING YOUR SLEEP EFFICIENCY

Starting with week 2 of your sleep program, you'll revise the amount of time you spend in bed each week (the amount that you restrict your sleep) based on your sleep efficiency the previous week. Remember, sleep efficiency is the percentage of time you're actually sleeping when you're in bed. At the end of each week of your sleep restriction program, calculate your sleep efficiency for that week by dividing your total sleep time (TST) by your total time in bed (TIB), then multiplying that number by 100. So if your average total sleep time is 5.3 hours and your total time in bed is 6 hours, your sleep efficiency is 88 percent (5.3 divided by 6, times 100).

The higher your sleep efficiency is, the better. A sleep efficiency over 90 percent is ideal, as that means you're spending less than 10 percent of your time in bed awake. For this sleep program, you should calculate your average sleep efficiency across the week. You can use either averages across the week or grand totals to do the calculations, whichever is easiest for you. Both methods result in the same number.

If your sleep efficiency is 90 percent or more for the week, you can increase the amount of time you spend in bed by 15 minutes the following week. If it's between 85 and 90 percent, your time in bed remains the same. If your sleep efficiency falls below 85 percent, you should decrease the amount of time you're allowed to spend in bed by 15 minutes. However, if you're already at the lower limit of 5 hours in bed each night, stick with 5 hours until you improve your sleep efficiency.

Here's an example of using sleep efficiency to determine the amount of time allowed in bed each night: Before starting sleep restriction, Karen kept her sleep log for a week and found that she averaged 5.5 hours of sleep each night (average TST). However, she spent an average of 8 hours in bed each night (average TIB). For week 1, her sleep efficiency was 69 percent. Since this is the first week of her sleep restriction program, her allowable time in bed is 5.5 hours each night, because that's her average TST. She set her bedtime at 12 midnight and her rise time at 5:30 a.m. For the next week she tried to follow the rules of stimulus control and get out of bed whenever she wasn't sleeping, but sometimes she felt so exhausted that she just stayed in bed.

For week 2, her average TST was 5 hours of sleep per night and her average TIB was 5.75 hours per night, so her sleep efficiency was 87 percent. Following the sleep restriction guidelines, Karen kept her sleep period the same for the next week, going to bed and getting up at the same time, and restricting herself to no more than 5.5 hours in bed each night.

For week 3, Karen's average TST was 5.25 hours and her average TIB was 5.5 hours, so her sleep efficiency increased to 95 percent. This is great! In just three weeks she's improved her sleep efficiency significantly and is getting more consolidated, solid sleep. Now she can increase her sleep period to 5.75 hours. Since starting the sleep restriction program, she's been quite sleepy at night and falls asleep quickly, so she moves her bedtime 15 minutes earlier, to 11:45 p.m. and keeps her rise time the same.

In week 4, Karen continues sleeping solidly. Her sleep efficiency is 92 percent, so she increases her time in bed by another 15 minutes, to 6 hours. Her bedtime is now 11:30 p.m. and her rise time is 5:30 a.m.

In week 5, she continues making progress. Her sleep efficiency is 95 percent, so she can increase her time in bed to 6.25 hours. Karen now sleeps from 11:30 p.m. to 5:45 a.m.

For week 6, Karen's sleep efficiency is 87 percent, so she keeps her sleep period the same for the next week. For weeks 7 and 8, her sleep efficiency is 95 percent, so she increases her sleep time by another 15 minutes each week. Now that she's getting 6.75 hours of solid sleep per night, Karen says she feels good during the day and doesn't think she needs more sleep. She's satisfied with her new sleep schedule, from 11:30 p.m. to 6:15 a.m.

Let's break down Karen's sleep in a week-by-week format, so you can clearly see how sleep restriction works when you calculate your sleep efficiency:

- *Week 1*: Sleep restriction based on average TST of 5.5 hours.

- *Week 2*: Based on a sleep efficiency (SE) of 87 percent in week 1, no changes are made to the sleep window. Sleep remains restricted to 5.5 hours each night.

- *Week 3*: SE is 95 percent, so 15 minutes are added to the sleep window, allowing 5.75 hours in bed each night.

- *Week 4*: SE is 92 percent. Another 15 minutes are added to the sleep window, allowing 6 hours in bed each night.

- *Week 5*: SE is 95 percent. Another 15 minutes are added to the sleep window, allowing 6.25 hours in bed each night.

- *Week 6*: SE is 87 percent, so the sleep window stays the same at 6.25 hours per night.

- *Week 7*: SE is 95 percent, so the sleep window is increased by 15 minutes, to 6.5 hours per night.

- *Week 8*: SE is 95 percent, so the sleep window is increased by another 15 minutes, allowing 6.75 in bed each night.

Sleep Restriction Worksheet for the Sleep Efficiency Method

You may find it helpful to have a worksheet to keep track of your sleep restriction program. To get started the first week, you just need to calculate your average total sleep time (average TST) over the previous week, to serve as the starting point for your allowable time in bed, or sleep window (SW). However, you may want to go ahead and calculate your sleep efficiency for the previous week as well, as it will provide a useful gauge of your progress. Choose a consistent bedtime and rise time for the next week based on your allowable time in bed. After week 1, calculate your sleep efficiency (SE) by dividing your average TST by your average time in bed (average TIB) and then multiplying by 100. On the next line, note whether you should increase your sleep window, decrease it, or keep it the same. As a reminder, you can increase your sleep window by 15 minutes if your sleep efficiency is 90 percent or greater. Decrease your sleep window by 15 minutes if your sleep efficiency is less than 85 percent (but don't restrict it to less than 5 hours). If your sleep efficiency is between 85 and 90 percent, keep your sleep window the same. Write down the number of hours in your newly calculated sleep window, along with your bedtime and rise time.

Week 1:   Average TST _____   Bedtime: _____   Rise time: _____

Week 2:   Average TST _____   Average TIB _____   SE _____

           Circle one: Increase SW   Decrease SW   Keep same SW

           Calculated SW _____   Bedtime: _____   Rise time: _____

Week 3:   Average TST _____   Average TIB _____   SE _____

           Circle one: Increase SW   Decrease SW   Keep same SW

           Calculated SW _____   Bedtime: _____   Rise time: _____

Week 4:   Average TST _____   Average TIB _____   SE _____

           Circle one: Increase SW   Decrease SW   Keep same SW

           Calculated SW _____   Bedtime: _____   Rise time: _____

Week 5:   Average TST _____   Average TIB _____   SE _____

           Circle one: Increase SW   Decrease SW   Keep same SW

           Calculated SW _____   Bedtime: _____   Rise time: _____

Week 6:   Average TST _____   Average TIB _____   SE _____

           Circle one: Increase SW   Decrease SW   Keep same SW

           Calculated SW _____   Bedtime: _____   Rise time: _____

Week 7:   Average TST _____   Average TIB _____   SE _____

           Circle one: Increase SW   Decrease SW   Keep same SW

           Calculated SW _____   Bedtime: _____   Rise time: _____

Week 8:   Average TST _____   Average TIB _____   SE _____

           Circle one: Increase SW   Decrease SW   Keep same SW

           Calculated SW _____   Bedtime: _____   Rise time: _____

ANOTHER OPTION FOR REVISING YOUR TIME IN BED: THE "SLEEPING SOLIDLY" APPROACH

Although calculating your sleep efficiency is the most precise way to implement sleep restriction, there's another method you can use to determine the amount of time you're allowed in bed each night. You still need to start by calculating your average TST based on at least a week of data in your sleep log, and you'll still restrict your time in bed to that number of hours the first week. How this approach differs is in how you determine whether you can increase or decrease the amount of time you're allowed in bed each night. Before you can increase it, you need to be sleeping solidly for one entire week. "Sleeping solidly" means that you don't wake up during the night, or if you do, you just wake up briefly and then fall back asleep in a couple of minutes.

Here's an example: John kept his sleep log for one week. Because he averaged 6 hours of sleep per night during week 1, he started restricting his time in bed to a total of 6 hours each night. After one week of restricted sleep, he still woke up several times each night. When that happened, he got up and engaged in boring or relaxing activities, and he also followed the other stimulus control guidelines to help form new, sleep-promoting associations between his bed and restful sleep. Since he still wasn't sleeping solidly through the night, he continued to restrict his sleep to 6 hours per night for week 3.

By the following week, he was sleeping solidly for the full 6 hours of his sleep window, falling asleep quickly and not waking up until his alarm clock rang the following morning. Because he was sleeping solidly during week 3, he increased his time in bed by 15 minutes, to 6.25 hours. Because he continued to sleep well during week 4, he increased his time in bed by another 15 minutes, to 6.5 hours. During weeks 5 and 6, John also slept solidly, so he increased his sleep by 15 minutes two more times. At that point, John was sleeping 7 hours per night and said that he felt rested and energetic during the day and didn't think he needed more sleep.

Let's break down John's sleep on a week-by-week basis, so you can clearly see how the sleeping solidly approach works:

- *Week 1:* Average TST of 6 hours.

- *Week 2:* Restricted sleep to 6 hours based on average TST. Frequent awakenings and not yet sleeping solidly. Continued sleep restriction of 6 hours per night.

- *Week 3:* Sleeping solidly. Increased sleep window to 6.25 hours per night.

- *Week 4:* Sleeping solidly. Increased sleep window to 6.5 hours per night.

- *Week 5:* Sleeping solidly. Increased sleep window to 6.75 hours per night.

- *Week 6:* Sleeping solidly. Increased sleep window to 7 hours per night.

Although this method of calculating your sleep window isn't as precise as using sleep efficiency, it certainly is easier, and it can be very effective if you stick to the stimulus control guidelines. So if you're lying awake during your sleep window, you need to get up out of bed and do something boring or relaxing until you feel sleepy, and you still need to get up at your scheduled rise time each day.

Sleep Restriction Worksheet Using the Sleeping Solidly Approach

Here's a worksheet you can use to design your sleep restriction program using the sleeping solidly approach. The first week, you just need to calculate your average total sleep time (average TST), to serve as the starting point for your allowable time in bed, or sleep window (SW). Set a consistent bedtime and rise time for the next week based on your allowable time in bed. At the end of week 2, assess whether you slept solidly every night. Be honest here, as the success of your sleep restriction program depends on an accurate answer. On the next line, note whether you should increase your sleep window, decrease it, or keep it the same. Write down the number of hours in your newly calculated sleep window, along with your bedtime and wake time.

Week 1:   Average TST _____   Bedtime: _____   Rise time: _____

Week 2:   Average TST _____   Are you sleeping solidly every night? ☐ yes ☐ no

          Circle one: Increase SW   Decrease SW   Keep same SW

          Bedtime: _____   Rise time: _____

Week 3:   Average TST _____   Are you sleeping solidly every night? ☐ yes ☐ no

          Circle one: Increase SW   Decrease SW   Keep same SW

          Bedtime: _____   Rise time: _____

Week 4:   Average TST _____   Are you sleeping solidly every night? ☐ yes ☐ no

          Circle one: Increase SW   Decrease SW   Keep same SW

          Bedtime: _____   Rise time: _____

Week 5:   Average TST _____   Are you sleeping solidly every night? ☐ yes ☐ no

          Circle one: Increase SW   Decrease SW   Keep same SW

          Bedtime: _____   Rise time: _____

Week 6:   Average TST _____   Are you sleeping solidly every night? ☐ yes ☐ no

          Circle one: Increase SW   Decrease SW   Keep same SW

          Bedtime: _____   Rise time: _____

Week 7:   Average TST _____   Are you sleeping solidly every night? ☐ yes ☐ no

Circle one: Increase SW   Decrease SW   Keep same SW

Bedtime: _____   Rise time: _____

Week 8:   Average TST _____   Are you sleeping solidly every night? ☐ yes ☐ no

Circle one: Increase SW   Decrease SW   Keep same SW

Bedtime: _____   Rise time: _____

Stick with the Program

If up to eight weeks seems like a long time to get yourself sleeping better, think about how long you've been sleeping poorly. All of those weeks, months, or years have ingrained some poor sleep habits, and it will take time to undo that conditioning. Many people are fortunate enough to feel better after just two or three weeks of sleep restriction and stimulus control, and hopefully this will be the case for you, as well. But remember, this sleep program is a process and isn't intended to be a quick-fix solution. If you're sleeping better after a couple of weeks, that's great news! But don't despair if it takes a little bit longer for you, and try to remember that these weeks are nothing in comparison with all of the sleepless nights you've already experienced.

SUMMING UP

Together, stimulus control and sleep restriction can play a major role in overcoming insomnia. Stimulus control works by changing the associations you have between not sleeping well and your bed, bedtime, or bedroom. By following some straightforward guidelines, you can replace these associations with new, more positive, sleep-promoting associations. So instead of feeling wide awake or keyed up when you get into bed at night, you'll be more likely to feel calm and sleepy. In addition, by limiting the amount of time you're allowed to be in bed each night with a sleep restriction program, you'll build up a sleep debt that will help you fall asleep easier. Sleep restriction also helps consolidate your sleep, so that the sleep you do get is deeper and more restorative. With time, sleep restriction will allow you to establish a regular sleep-wake schedule that works well for you.

CHAPTER 8

Controlling Anxiety and Irrational Thoughts

Suzanne is plagued by anxious thoughts. She worries about her job, her kids, her health, and, of course, her sleep. She lies awake most nights thinking about all of the things she has to do and feeling overwhelmed. But her anxious thoughts aren't just keeping her up at night, they disturb her during the day as well. Even when she's in the middle of a fun activity with friends or family, she can easily become consumed by her thoughts. Sometimes it starts out innocently enough, just thinking about her day or something someone said to her. But the thoughts start becoming more negative, irrational, and relentless. Soon she finds herself feeling like she's drowning in a glass of water, as what started out as a simple passing thought takes on a life of its own and fills her with more anxiety and dread, and she feels powerless to stop it. Suzanne isn't sure where to turn next, but she knows that she can't continue feeling so anxious all the time.

In chapters 4 through 7, I focused on the behavioral components of this sleep program, discussing various behaviors that contribute to poor sleep and how to change them. You've learned about sleep hygiene, relaxation techniques, how to record your sleep in a sleep log, and how to implement stimulus control and sleep restriction. You may be sleeping better already. However, some people experience anxiety along with their sleep problems, which makes insomnia worse. If that's the case for you, as it was for Suzanne, you can benefit from learning the skills in this chapter, which will help you control your anxiety and decrease irrational thoughts and cognitive distortions.

COGNITIVE DISTORTIONS

Dysfunctional beliefs, or cognitive distortions, can play a major role in anxiety. You may have various types of distorted thoughts, including all-or-nothing thinking, overgeneralization, catastrophic thinking, negative automatic thoughts, and jumping to conclusions. Let's take a look at these types of cognitive distortions, which can make your anxiety, and therefore your sleep, worse.

All-or-Nothing Thinking

Thinking in an all-or-nothing way is thinking in absolute terms, using words such as "never," "every," or "always." For example, if you say, "I'll never be as good as my brother" or "I always screw up when making presentations at work," you're thinking in an all-or-nothing way. This is a cognitive distortion, because life isn't usually so absolute. All-or-nothing thinking can make you feel more anxious or depressed, and it can cause you to make decisions that aren't based in logic. When you realize that things aren't so black and white and that you have more options available to you, you can start to see and think a bit differently.

For example, if you're unhappy in a relationship, all-or-nothing thinking may lead you to jump to a conclusion such as "I've never been happy in this relationship and things will never get better. I need to get out of it quickly and never see this person again." This is a fairly drastic example, and although some situations may actually be that bad, it's unlikely that you were *never* happy in the relationship, or that things could *never* get better in the future. After all, why would you have gotten in the relationship if it had never been good? Can you remember a time when things were better? What was different about the relationship then? What about trying to work on the relationship together? What other options are there? Thinking you need to leave the situation and never see the person again is a very absolute solution. Instead, perhaps you need a little break from the relationship, or perhaps you should try couples counseling. When you think in all-or-nothing terms, you won't consider all of your options and therefore may suffer harsher consequences in the future.

All-or-Nothing Thinking Worksheet

During the day, use the following worksheet to record all-or-nothing statements that go through your head or that you notice yourself saying out loud. For each, come up with some alternative ways of thinking. Here's an example, followed by a blank worksheet you can copy if you like.

Date	All-or-Nothing Thinking	Alternative Ways of Thinking
3/15	*I'll never improve my status at work.*	*I've already been told by my boss that I'm doing well, so that's a good sign. Perhaps I can speak with him about improving my status at work.*

| 3/17 | I always procrastinate, and there's nothing I can do about it. | I can start to write down a list of things I need to do and make a schedule for doing them. Also, when it's something that I really like to do, I don't tend to procrastinate at all. |

Date	All-or-Nothing Thinking	Alternative Ways of Thinking

Overgeneralization

Making wide generalizations from isolated, specific cases is called overgeneralization. Like all-or-nothing thinking, this type of cognitive distortion can increase your anxiety. Let's say a supervisor at work tells you that you made a mistake on a project you're working on. It's human. Everyone makes mistakes. But if you were to take that one specific mistake and generalize it to other situations, your thinking might go something like this: "I made a mistake at work today. I'm no good at my job, and my boss must think I'm an idiot." This is an irrational, overgeneralized response. Instead, you could think, "I made a mistake at work today. It happens. I don't usually make these kinds of mistakes, so I'll learn from it and try to do better next time." Not only is the first way of thinking an overgeneralization, it's also filled with negative thinking. The second line of thought is more rational, specific, and objective. When you restructure your thoughts to acknowledge the details and complexity of a situation, you can find more appropriate solutions to problems and not get stuck in a pattern of negativity.

Overgeneralization Worksheet

During the day, use the following worksheet to record instances of overgeneralization that go through your head or that you notice yourself saying out loud. For each, come up with some alternative ways of thinking. Here's an example, followed by a blank worksheet you can copy if you like.

Date	Overgeneralization	Alternative Ways of Thinking
8/15	*My child hit another kid at school today. This is a sign that he's going to be aggressive and difficult to manage for his entire life. What a problem.*	*This is the first time my child has ever hit another kid. He was upset and sorry about it afterward and said he wouldn't do it again. He was also sad because another kid was teasing him. He just needs to learn other ways to deal with his frustration.*
8/17	*I just broke up with my boyfriend and I'm never going to find someone else. I'll be single and alone forever.*	*It's a hard time right now because I just broke up with my boyfriend. But it happens to other people, too, and they manage to survive. Just because it didn't work out this time doesn't mean that I'll never find someone.*

Date	Overgeneralization	Alternative Ways of Thinking

Catastrophic Thinking

Another cognitive distortion that can lead to anxiety is catastrophic thinking, or catastrophizing, in which you exaggerate, or magnify, the importance of certain events or experiences and predict the worst possible outcome. In this type of thinking, the positive characteristics of others may be exaggerated, while their negative characteristics are ignored or minimized. The same holds true for situations that occur regularly. For example, let's say you go to the doctor for some headaches you've been having recently. The doctor tells you that it's probably nothing, but he wants to do a few tests just to make sure. If you start catastrophizing, you might exaggerate the situation in your mind, thinking, "Run a few tests?! Why would the doctor run a few tests unless he thinks I have something really serious? I bet I have cancer…maybe a brain tumor. I'll probably be dead before my fiftieth birthday." This is catastrophic thinking because most headaches don't result in cancer or a serious illness. The headaches could be related to stress or many other things, but if you engage in catastrophic thinking, you'll fear the worst, and this will create unnecessary stress and anxiety in your life.

DO YOU MAKE MOUNTAINS OUT OF MOLEHILLS?

Catastrophic thinking involves making mountains out of molehills, which can definitely increase your anxiety and make it more difficult for you to fall asleep at night. Here's an example: Let's say you get into a minor car accident, where only your left rear taillight needs replacing. No one is hurt, and all things considered, the situation is pretty good. But instead of remembering those positive details, you focus only on the negative and the situation takes on a life of its own. You think, "I'll go to the mechanic, and he'll probably charge me a fortune to replace the taillight. Plus, my insurance rates will go up. I bet there will be a report in the paper and everyone will find out about it. I'll probably get sued for damages, and they'll try to take my house away."

Clearly, you've magnified a minor event into a major catastrophe, and it's all occurring in your head. Even if some of the thoughts might be true (like your insurance rates may go up or it may be expensive to replace the taillight), you're making much more out of them than the situation calls for, which leads to more anxiety and frustration. In addition to adding to your daytime level of stress, this way of thinking can cause anxiety that keeps you up at night, so it's important to put a stop to it.

HOW CATASTROPHIC THINKING IMPACTS SLEEP

If you tend to think the worst will probably happen in most situations, your catastrophic thinking is probably affecting many aspects of your life, including your sleep. For example, when you're having a bad night of sleep, you may think, "I'm not getting enough sleep tonight, so I'm going to be a wreck at work tomorrow. I won't be productive, and I'll be in a bad mood. My coworkers will tell my boss about my poor performance, and I may get fired. It's going to be a horrible, unbearable day if I don't get enough sleep." Although these thoughts may make sense in a way, they're actually irrational because there have probably been many times when you didn't sleep well and yet still were productive at work. Maybe you didn't feel as great as other days, but you weren't necessarily in a bad mood or especially prone to making errors. Catastrophic thinking can make an uncomfortable situation feel unbearable or impossible. Although you may not feel your best after a bad night of sleep, dwelling on it and focusing on the worst possible outcome only makes the situation seem worse. It increases your anxiety and makes it hard to focus on other things—and it probably leads to an even worse night of sleep than you would have had without catastrophic thinking.

Catastrophic Thinking Worksheet

Use the following worksheet to record times when you engage in catastrophic thinking. Record all of your catastrophic thoughts associated with the situation, and then think of some alternative ways of thinking about the situation. By writing down alternative responses, you can replace your catastrophic thinking with a more realistic assessment, which will help decrease your anxiety. Here's an example, followed by a blank worksheet you can copy if you like.

Date	Catastrophic Thinking	Alternative Ways of Thinking
6/15	When I was at work today, I asked a colleague for help with my computer. She probably thinks that I'm stupid because I don't know what I'm doing. I felt embarrassed and upset that she knows so much more than me.	Everybody needs help sometimes. My colleague was very nice to me and showed me how to fix the problem. She said that she has the same computer problem sometimes and that it happens to everyone.
6/16	Tonight at a party, I slipped and fell in front of a bunch of people. I felt like a klutz. I'm so clumsy and dumb. Everyone must have thought I was the biggest loser there.	The floor was wet, which is why I fell. People asked me if I was okay afterward, so they must have cared about how I was doing. I don't typically fall, and in general I'm not very clumsy, so I shouldn't feel so bad about it.

Date	Catastrophic Thinking	Alternative Ways of Thinking

Negative Automatic Thoughts

People with anxiety or depression typically have negative automatic thoughts throughout the day. In general, these are the thoughts or images that surface during times of stress or disappointment. For example, if you're concerned about what others think of you, you may have negative thoughts like "They don't like my clothes" or "They probably think I don't know what I'm talking about" when you're with a group of people. This negative way of thinking affects the way you interact with other people, how you view the world around you, and how you view the future. By starting to identify your negative thoughts, you can begin to change them to more positive thoughts. This can help you have more positive interactions with others and a more optimistic view of the world around you and the future.

IS YOUR GLASS HALF EMPTY OR HALF FULL?

If you frequently experience negative automatic thoughts, they could be significantly diminishing your quality of life. When you see most things with a negative spin, it can be hard to work your way out of the negativity, especially because negative thoughts can influence your emotions. For example, if you have a negative thought about a health concern, you may feel intense anxiety, which will elevate your heart rate, and when you feel this, you may think it's a cause for concern. Later, while exercising, you may interpret your pounding heart as a sign that you may be having a heart attack, so you'll feel even more anxious and upset. You'll probably stop exercising and dwell on your negative thoughts. As a result, your life becomes more limited and your health may actually become a genuine concern. In addition, negative thoughts can affect your memory and concentration, which can certainly cause even more upsetting thoughts (Fennell 1998). Thinking negatively can also make you feel helpless, as though there's nothing you can do to change the situation or make it better. But this isn't true; there's almost always something you can do to improve any situation. A good place to start is by changing your negative thoughts and starting to think more positively.

HOW NEGATIVE THOUGHTS CAN AFFECT YOUR LIFE

Negative thoughts can affect your behaviors, how you get along with other people, and how you react to situations. For example, let's say you have to give a presentation at work tomorrow. You're well prepared, having gone over your notes many times. You've even rehearsed your presentation in front of your spouse. When you get to work the next day, you realize that you forgot to bring along a handout that you thought might be useful. You really don't need it for the presentation, but if your negative thoughts kick in, here's what you may be thinking: "I'm useless. I can't do anything right. I forgot that handout, and now it will ruin my presentation. Nothing will ever get any better."

Negative thoughts can impact your relationships as well. It's hard to be around someone who's always negative about life. Imagine this scenario: You're out having dinner at a new restaurant. You've just ordered your meal, when you notice that you spilled some water on your shirt. You know it won't stain, but your negative thinking makes you feel awful. You think, "I am so clumsy. I'm pathetic. I can never go anywhere without looking like a fool. This has ruined my night. I don't know why I even bother." Now, rather than enjoying a nice evening out, you're dwelling on the negative aspects. Even if you don't actually express any of your thoughts out loud, you're still thinking them, so they're affecting your mood. Others will pick up on this, so it will impact their evening as well. Not only will you feel badly, but others may not know what to do to help.

If you tend to see the negative in situations and in other people, automatically assume the worst in stressful situations, or dwell on one negative event even when positive events have also occurred, you engage in negative thinking. Fortunately, you can change the way you think. As with changing all-or-nothing thinking or catastrophic thinking, you can come up with alternative thoughts, which will improve your mood and emotions—and probably your sleep.

Negative Thinking Worksheet

Use the following worksheet to help you start identifying your negative thoughts and the emotions related to them, and alternative ways of thinking about the situation. First record the date, then describe the situation: exactly what happened that led to your negative thoughts. Next, list the emotions you felt as a result of the situation and rate them on a scale of 0 to 10, with 10 being a very strong emotion. Next, describe your negative thoughts and rate how much you believe them, from 0 to 100 percent. So if you put 90 percent, you strongly believe that negative thought is true. Next, come up with alternative, more rational responses and rate how much you believe them, again from 0 to 100 percent. See if these alternative thoughts help change your emotions or their strength. Here's an example, followed by a blank worksheet you can copy if you like.

Date	Situation	Emotions (0-10)	Negative Automatic Thoughts (0-100%)	Alternative Thoughts (0-100%)
5/5	I was at the supermarket and realized I forgot my wallet.	Anxious: 8 Sad: 5 Angry: 6	I'm such an idiot. I'm so forgetful and disorganized. I'm embarrassed and can never show up at this supermarket again. 90%	Everyone forgets things once in a while. 50% I rushed out of the house to pick up the kids from school and then headed to the store. I was running late, so it makes sense that I forgot it. 80% I'm usually pretty organized, and this is the first time I've done this. 75%

Date	Situation	Emotions (0-10)	Negative Automatic Thoughts (0-100%)	Alternative Thoughts (0-100%)

Jumping to Conclusions

Another cognitive distortion that can cause anxiety in your life is jumping to conclusions. This means that you assume that something is going to happen (usually something negative) before you have sufficient evidence to support that conclusion. Variations on this type of thinking include fortune-telling, or predicting how a situation will turn out before it happens, and mind reading, or assuming you know what other people are thinking. Both involve jumping to conclusions too quickly, and with mind reading, you aren't allowing others a chance to express themselves. For example, say you're at work and have a question for your supervisor. But you're nervous about asking because you assume your supervisor will get annoyed at you and think you don't know what you're doing. However, by not asking the question, you're actually increasing your anxiety because you'll feel less sure about what you're doing. So you're the one who suffers in this situation. Your supervisor may or may not get annoyed at you for asking, but that really isn't something you can know in advance. The only way you'll know for sure is to go ahead and ask so you can actually see your supervisor's reaction.

Here's another example of jumping to conclusions: You're waiting for an appointment at the doctor's office. You've signed in and notice that a couple of people who showed up after you went in first. If you start jumping to conclusions, you could assume that the office staff don't like you and are purposely letting others go before you (mind reading). Then you might jump to another conclusion and assume your doctor is going to drop you as a patient (fortune telling). A better approach than jumping to conclusions is to simply ask the office staff about it. Perhaps the other people had earlier appointments and the office goes by appointment time, not when you arrive at the office. Or perhaps the other patients had medical emergencies and needed to be seen right away. In any case, there's no evidence that your doctor would drop you as a patient, which seems like a very unlikely outcome. Doctors' offices are busy and it's often necessary to wait. It may be annoying, but it's usually nothing personal.

In addition, making assumptions before you have all of the facts available can impair your relationships with others. If you think you know what other people are thinking or what their intentions are, you probably don't feel the need to ask them directly. This can lead to a whole assortment of problems. For example, imagine that you're on the phone with a friend and suddenly you notice a small fire in the kitchen. You don't have time to explain what's going on, so you simply say, "I'll call you back," and hang up. If your friend starts jumping to conclusions, she might think, "Gee, she must have gotten upset when I mentioned that party I went to on Saturday night. I didn't know she wasn't invited. I shouldn't have said anything. Now she's mad at me and won't want to be my friend anymore."

Jumping to conclusions can cause considerable anxiety in situations where it's completely unnecessary. In the example above, perhaps you didn't care at all about not being invited to the party because you're not close friends with the host. In addition, you really value your friendship and wouldn't let something so silly get in the way. But by short-circuiting the process of talking about these things out loud, your friend has jumped to conclusions that could lead to hurt feelings, misunderstandings, and added stress. Next time you notice you're heading in that direction, simply stop yourself and try to get more information. Once you have all of the facts, you can make better decisions based in reality, not just what's going on in your head.

Jumping to Conclusions Worksheet

Use the following worksheet to record your thoughts in situations where you jump to conclusions. If you're assuming you know other people's thoughts or intentions, designate those thoughts MR, for mind reading. If you're predicting how things will turn out, designate those thoughts FT, for fortune telling. Then write down some alternative ways of thinking about the situation. Here's an example, followed by a blank worksheet you can copy if you like.

Date	Jumping to Conclusions	Alternative Ways of Thinking
7/15	When I arrived at work today, some of my colleagues were gathered together. They were probably talking about me, saying rude things. (MR)	My colleagues did ask me how I was doing and they're usually pretty friendly. I haven't noticed that they talk about other people behind their backs, so I shouldn't just jump to conclusions.
7/16	My boss left a message for me to see him at the end of the day. He probably thinks my last project wasn't good enough. Maybe he wants to fire me. (MR/FT)	Maybe my boss does want to discuss my last project—to tell me what a great job I did. Or maybe he just wants to see how things are going for me. There's no way I can know, so I'll wait until our meeting and not jump to any conclusions.

Date	Jumping to Conclusions	Alternative Ways of Thinking

COUNTERING COGNITIVE DISTORTIONS

With all of these cognitive distortions, your thoughts may sound logical and plausible, but they typically aren't rational. With catastrophizing, for example, you're expecting the worst possible outcome even though it's quite unlikely that it will actually occur. In the exercises above, you've worked on coming up with alternative ways of thinking. This sort of brainstorming will help you see other possibilities. The next step in banishing cognitive distortions, or at least weakening them, is to weigh the evidence for and against your thoughts. If your thoughts stem from your own fears and negative self-talk, you're likely to find that there isn't much evidence to support them. By becoming aware of any tendency to make conclusions that aren't based on evidence, you can start thinking more rationally and decrease unnecessary anxiety.

Let's take a closer look at how to examine the evidence for and against something actually happening. For example, let's say you're driving in your car and hear a funny noise that lasts for about one second. As you continue driving, you start to fear that your car is broken in some way. Maybe you have a flat tire, or maybe your engine is about to die. You feel your heart beating faster and your breathing becoming more rapid as your mind fills with negative thoughts about your ability to cope with these feared possibilities. When you notice anxiety setting in, you need to examine the evidence for and against your fears.

For: I heard a funny noise that lasted about one second. Funny noises in cars can mean problems.

Against: The car still seems to be driving fine. Perhaps I went over a bump in the road or over some debris. I took the car in for a routine tune-up last week, and the mechanic said everything was fine. So it probably isn't a mechanical problem. There's no obvious reason why my engine would die, and if it were a flat tire, I would feel it while I'm driving. Instead, everything seems to be okay.

In this example, there seems to be much more evidence against the fear than for it. What do you think the probability is that either of these fears is realistic? In reality, it's actually very low, probably well under 10 percent.

It's also worthwhile to look at your ability to cope with the things you fear. Having a more realistic assessment of your ability to cope with the worst possible scenario can take some of the charge out of the situation. In this case, you might tell yourself, "It's so unlikely that the engine would actually die. My car is only two years old and it was just serviced last week. Even getting a flat tire, which is much more common, wouldn't be that bad. I did get a flat tire while driving one time. I was very nervous, but I managed to safely pull over to the side of the road and call for help. So if that were to happen, I could just call a local garage or a friend for help, or even try to fix it on my own. I coped pretty well last time I got a flat tire, so there's no reason to believe that this time would be any worse.

Irrational Thoughts Worksheet

The following worksheet will help you assess the likelihood of your fears coming true and allow you to explore your ability to cope if what you fear were to actually occur. First, describe the situation that caused you to start feeling anxious. Next, write what you fear will happen. In the next two columns, record the evidence for and against your fear actually coming true. Take some time to weigh the evidence for and against, and then assign a percentage to how realistic it is that the feared event will occur. Finally, imagine that what you fear does actually occur, and assess your ability to cope with the situation.

Situation	What You Fear Will Happen	Evidence for the Feared Event Occurring	Evidence Against the Feared Event Occurring	Realistic Probability (0-100%)	Assessment of Your Ability to Cope
Driving in my car and I heard a noise.	I'll get a flat tire or my engine will die.	Flat tires can happen at any time, and I've had flat tires in the past.	My car was just serviced and there were no problems. I was able to keep driving and it didn't feel like anything was wrong with the car. Little noises happen in cars sometimes, even when there's nothing wrong. If the tire was flat, I would have felt it, and I'd know if the engine died because the car would stop working.	Less than 5%.	I could cope with a flat tire, as I've managed in the past. I could call a friend, go to a garage, or even fix it myself. Overall, I could handle the situation pretty well.

Situation	What You Fear Will Happen	Evidence for the Feared Event Occurring	Evidence Against the Feared Event Occurring	Realistic Probability (0-100%)	Assessment of Your Ability to Cope

RACING THOUGHTS

Another thinking pattern that can worsen anxiety is racing thoughts. This refers to thoughts that just won't stop. They can be about nearly anything: the things you did during the day, conversations you had, music you heard, something you saw on television, various worries, and so on. These thoughts occur rapidly and aren't inhibited. In other words, they just keep coming. If this is an issue for you, there are a couple of techniques you can try to calm your mind: distraction techniques and thought stopping.

Distraction Techniques

There are a number of different types of distraction techniques you can try when you have racing thoughts, including thinking of good memories, doing mental exercises, engaging in absorbing activities, focusing on a particular object, and increasing your sensory awareness (Fennell 1998). Let's take a look at each of these.

Thinking of good memories can help decrease racing thoughts and anxiety. Think back on positive memories from the past, like a fun party or a great vacation and think of how much fun you had and how relaxed and happy you felt. Really focus on the details: Where were you? Who else was there? Do you remember lots of laughing and smiling? You can also think of a good movie that you've seen. Try to remember the names of the characters, the different scenes, and so on. Or you can think of a book you recently enjoyed. Whatever subject you choose, try to remember the details.

Doing mental exercises can be helpful because you have to focus your thoughts to do them. For example, try thinking of as many countries or cities that start with the letter A as you can. Next try the letter S, and so on. Pick any letter and concentrate on the task. Alternatively, you can count to one hundred going up by threes or do math calculations in your head. Another idea is to try to recall the lyrics of some of your favorite songs. Whenever you focus on these sorts of mental exercises, you won't be able to get so caught up in or overwhelmed by anxious or racing thoughts.

Engaging in absorbing activities involves activities that occupy both your mind and your body (Fennell 1998). For example, you can do Sudoku, crossword puzzles, or more physical activities. Certain types of exercise don't occupy your mind as much, so they won't be as helpful in stopping racing thoughts. For example, swimming and jogging tend to be more monotonous activities that don't require much mental concentration. But sports that require you to actively think, like tennis, basketball, squash, or soccer, can be helpful. Working out with an exercise video is also a good choice, because it occupies both your mind and your body. Having to pay attention to the video and follow along with the exercises can help decrease racing thoughts.

Focusing on a particular object involves devoting all of your attention on one specific object. Give yourself a detailed description of the object: What is it? What color is it? Where is it? What is it used for? How big or small is it? Does it have a smell? What is it made of? The possibilities for how to describe it are almost endless. Focusing on an object in this way is especially helpful for decreasing racing thoughts when you find yourself in an anxiety-provoking situation.

Increasing your sensory awareness involves focusing on your surroundings using all of your senses: taste, touch, smell, sound, and sight. Try to become very aware of what's going on around you and with your own body. Try sitting down in a chair then taking a look around you. What do you see? What do you hear? How does your body feel? Do you taste anything? Smell anything? Grounding yourself in your senses and your surroundings in this way may help calm your racing thoughts and anxiety, and you can do it anywhere and in almost any situation.

Thought Stopping

The idea behind thought stopping is to stop anxious, disturbing, or racing thoughts while they're occurring. There are two different techniques. Try both and see which works best for you. Here's the first technique: The next time a distressing thought enters your head, say, "*Stop!*" either to yourself or out loud. Picture a big red stop sign in your head at the same time. For at least a couple of seconds, the upsetting thought should go away. After saying "stop," try to think of an alternative positive thought instead (like a peaceful scene or something fun you did recently). The second technique for thought stopping involves wearing a rubber band on your wrist. Whenever an intrusive or disturbing thought enters your head, snap the rubber band against your wrist. Again, picturing a stop sign when you do this can help. Like the first technique, this one can stop the disturbing thought, at least temporarily. After you snap the rubber band, try to come up with an alternative, positive thought to replace the upsetting one.

SLEEP-RELATED FEARS AND DYSFUNCTIONAL BELIEFS

People have many different types of fears: fear of dying, fear of losing control, fear of being embarrassed in front of others, fear of illness, fear of losing a loved one, and many, many more. You may have other fears as well, perhaps related to your children, parents, friends, or financial situation—and, of course, your sleep. While fear can be a natural reaction to certain situations and circumstances, it can also stem from insecurity or uncertainty about the future. Whatever the cause, fears can certainly make you feel anxious and worried, and they can take on a life of their own and have a negative impact on your life.

If you don't deal with your fears, they can stop you from doing things or from enjoying many aspects of your life. As you learned in the previous exercise, it's important to consider whether your fears are based in reality. Is there evidence to support them? Examining your fears will help decrease your overall anxiety, and this will probably help improve your sleep.

In addition, it's important to evaluate your beliefs about sleep to see whether they're making your insomnia worse. For example, do you have unrealistic expectations about your sleep? Do you think you must get eight hours of sleep at night to function properly the next day? If you do, it would be helpful to look at the evidence behind that thought, just like you examined the evidence for and against certain fears in the previous exercise.

The way you think about your sleep definitely affects your mood and behaviors. For example, if you believe that getting a poor night of sleep will impair your performance at work the next day, you may become angry, irritable, or anxious just thinking about it. If you're having these thoughts and feelings in the middle of the night, they can keep you awake. If you carry this belief with you to work the next day, you're likely to feel frustrated and upset at work, even if your performance is perfectly fine. Similarly, if you start worrying about your sleep after dinner and predict that you'll have another bad night, you may feel helpless, out of control, anxious, or apprehensive (Morin 1993). These feelings can make your sleep problem worse that night. Who knows, maybe you wouldn't have had any trouble sleeping if you didn't start worrying about it first. Keep in mind that your emotions impact your behaviors, including your ability to fall asleep and stay asleep.

Dysfunctional Beliefs and Attitudes about Sleep (DBAS)

To assess your dysfunctional beliefs and attitudes about sleep, fill out the following questionnaire about common sleep-related beliefs, created by Dr. Charles Morin (1993).

Several statements reflecting people's beliefs and attitudes about sleep are listed below. Please indicate to what extent you personally agree or disagree with each statement. There is no right or wrong answer. For each statement, circle the number that corresponds to your own *personal belief*. Please respond to all items even though some may not apply directly to your own situation:

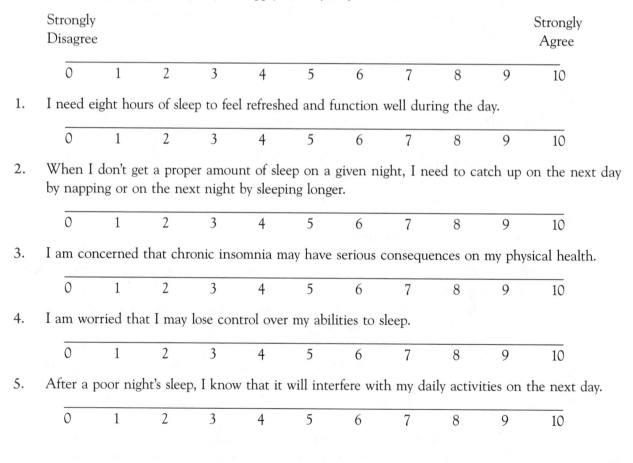

Strongly
Disagree

Strongly
Agree

| 0 | 1 | 2 | 3 | 4 | 5 | 6 | 7 | 8 | 9 | 10 |

1. I need eight hours of sleep to feel refreshed and function well during the day.

| 0 | 1 | 2 | 3 | 4 | 5 | 6 | 7 | 8 | 9 | 10 |

2. When I don't get a proper amount of sleep on a given night, I need to catch up on the next day by napping or on the next night by sleeping longer.

| 0 | 1 | 2 | 3 | 4 | 5 | 6 | 7 | 8 | 9 | 10 |

3. I am concerned that chronic insomnia may have serious consequences on my physical health.

| 0 | 1 | 2 | 3 | 4 | 5 | 6 | 7 | 8 | 9 | 10 |

4. I am worried that I may lose control over my abilities to sleep.

| 0 | 1 | 2 | 3 | 4 | 5 | 6 | 7 | 8 | 9 | 10 |

5. After a poor night's sleep, I know that it will interfere with my daily activities on the next day.

| 0 | 1 | 2 | 3 | 4 | 5 | 6 | 7 | 8 | 9 | 10 |

6.   In order to be alert and function well during the day, I believe I would be better off taking a sleeping pill rather than having a poor night's sleep.

0   1   2   3   4   5   6   7   8   9   10

7.   When I feel irritable, depressed, or anxious during the day, it's mostly because I didn't sleep well the night before.

0   1   2   3   4   5   6   7   8   9   10

8.   When I sleep poorly on one night, I know it will disturb my sleep schedule for the whole week.

0   1   2   3   4   5   6   7   8   9   10

9.   Without an adequate night's sleep, I can hardly function the next day.

0   1   2   3   4   5   6   7   8   9   10

10.   I can't ever predict whether I'll have a good or poor night's sleep.

0   1   2   3   4   5   6   7   8   9   10

11.   I have little ability to manage the negative consequences of disturbed sleep.

0   1   2   3   4   5   6   7   8   9   10

12.   When I feel tired, have no energy, or just seem not to function well during the day, it's generally because I didn't sleep well the night before.

0   1   2   3   4   5   6   7   8   9   10

13.   I believe insomnia is essentially the result of a chemical imbalance.

0   1   2   3   4   5   6   7   8   9   10

14.   I feel insomnia is ruining my ability to enjoy life and prevents me from doing what I want.

0   1   2   3   4   5   6   7   8   9   10

15.   Medication is probably the only solution to sleeplessness.

0   1   2   3   4   5   6   7   8   9   10

16.   I avoid or cancel obligations (social, family) after a poor night's sleep.

0   1   2   3   4   5   6   7   8   9   10

Did you find yourself agreeing with many of the statements in the DBAS? If so, you have some dysfunctional beliefs regarding your sleep. This means that the way you're thinking about your sleep is probably quite negative, and therefore making your sleep worse. In order to help you change these beliefs, let's take a close look at the problematic thinking involved in each statement.

Belief 1 states, "I need eight hours of sleep to feel refreshed and function well during the day." If you agree with that statement, you have a dysfunctional belief about the number of hours of sleep you need each night. As discussed, many people need less than eight hours of sleep to feel refreshed and function well during the day, and some people need more. Because sleep needs are individualized, it isn't possible to make a generalized statement like this. Consider whether there have been nights when you slept six or seven hours and still felt fine and functioned well the next day. Don't hold on to a false belief that you absolutely need eight hours of sleep. This only leads to more anxiety about sleep and can worsen your sleep problem.

Belief 2 states, "When I don't get a proper amount of sleep on a given night, I need to catch up on the next day by napping or on the next night by sleeping longer." If you agree with this statement, you believe that you need to catch up on sleep after a bad night. However, taking naps can actually make your sleep problem worse, since you only need a certain amount of sleep across a twenty-four-hour period. Similarly, allowing yourself to sleep longer than usual the following night may make it harder for you to fall asleep the next night. It's better to stick to the same sleep-wake schedule, regardless of how many hours of sleep you got the night before.

Belief 3 states, "I am concerned that chronic insomnia may have serious consequences on my physical health." This isn't exactly a dysfunctional belief, as chronic sleep deprivation can lead to health consequences. However, most people with insomnia spend too much time worrying about issues like this, which only makes their sleep problem worse. Instead of worrying about possible health consequences, it's a better idea to focus on ways to decrease your anxiety and thereby improve your overall sleep, and your health along with it.

Belief 4 states, "I am worried that I may lose control over my abilities to sleep." If you agree with this statement, you probably don't believe that you're in control of your sleep. However, your behaviors and actions do affect your sleep. If you think that you could lose control over your own ability to sleep, this implies that what you do or think during the day doesn't affect your sleep and that, in the end, it's out of your control. This simply isn't true. You are in control of your sleep, and making positive behavioral changes and decreasing your anxiety level can help you sleep better at night.

Belief 5 states, "After a poor night's sleep, I know that it will interfere with my daily activities on the next day." While you may feel a bit more tired the next day, you're probably still able to function and get through the day. In fact, many people with insomnia deny that their daytime functioning is impaired. Although it varies from person to person and depending on the circumstances, it isn't a good idea to dwell on this belief. Thinking that your activities will be affected the next day makes it likely that you'll be more self-conscious and aware of everything you do. Although you may be frustrated by a poor night of sleep, you can probably still manage just fine the next day. It's best not to ruminate on this too much.

Belief 6 states, "In order to be alert and function well during the day, I believe I would be better off taking a sleeping pill rather than having a poor night's sleep." However, because sleeping pills can actually cause you to have a hangover effect, you may feel more drowsy and groggy the next day, rather than more alert. In addition, many studies have shown that sleeping pills can actually decrease your performance and functioning the next day, so if you believe you'll do better with sleeping pills, you may want to think again. And remember, a sleeping pill doesn't always equal a good night of sleep, so it's important to weigh the pros and cons when considering whether to take a sleeping pill.

Belief 7 states, "When I feel irritable, depressed, or anxious during the day, it's mostly because I didn't sleep well the night before." If you agree with this belief, you are putting too much emphasis on the effects of a bad night's sleep on your mood. Although lack of sleep can contribute to feeling irritable, depressed, or anxious during the day, many other factors can be responsible for these feelings. Specific daytime events may be the cause, or you may have an independent mood disorder, one that's unrelated to your sleep disturbance. In the latter case, you may feel irritable, depressed, or anxious regardless of the number of hours you slept the night before. If you really think about it, you'll probably be able to come up with a number of other reasons for feeling irritable, anxious, or depressed.

Belief 8 states, "When I sleep poorly on one night, I know it will disturb my sleep schedule for the whole week." Sleeping poorly on one night need not disturb your sleep schedule for the rest of the week, and if you agree with the belief that it will, you're catastrophizing the situation. Instead, you can use a poor night of sleep as a signal that you need to take control of your sleep for the rest of the week. That means following good sleep hygiene, incorporating relaxation exercises on a daily basis, sticking to your sleep-wake schedule, and following the stimulus control guidelines, such as not allowing yourself to lie in bed for more than fifteen minutes when you feel wide awake. Overcoming your insomnia is a process that you're actively involved in, and there's no need to believe that one night of poor sleep will ruin the rest of your week.

Belief 9 states, "Without an adequate night's sleep, I can hardly function the next day." Similar to other dysfunctional beliefs in this questionnaire, agreeing with this belief means that you're probably exaggerating the effects of a bad night of sleep. You can probably still function fine the next day, and obsessing about it in your head will only make you feel worse. Try to remember all of the times when you've functioned just fine after a poor night of sleep. What's the evidence that you can't manage to do it again?

Belief 10 states, "I can't ever predict whether I'll have a good or poor night's sleep." If you agree with this belief, you probably haven't started keeping a sleep log yet. When you keep a sleep log, you'll see that there are often reasons why you have a good night versus a bad night. Once you learn what makes your sleep better or worse, you can begin to make changes that will promote better sleep.

Belief 11 states, "I have little ability to manage the negative consequences of disturbed sleep." This dysfunctional belief reflects a feeling that you have little or no control over your actions or thoughts during the day. However, you are in control of your day, and you can manage the consequences of a bad night of sleep. When you think there's nothing you can do, you feel helpless. As a result, you may not even try to do anything about the situation. A better approach is to remember that you are able to manage the consequences of a bad night of sleep, along with other stress in your life. (Chapter 9 offers guidance on dealing with daytime stress.)

Belief 12 states, "When I feel tired, have no energy, or just seem not to function well during the day, it's generally because I didn't sleep well the night before." There may be multiple reasons why you feel tired, lack energy, or don't function as well during the day. Not all are related to your sleep. For example, if you're sick, this can affect your stamina and how you feel during the day. Similarly, if you worked very hard the day before, with no breaks and little downtime, you may still feel worn out from that. Certain medications can also affect energy level, as can the food that you eat. In addition, sitting for prolonged periods can make you feel tired, so you may just need to get up and move around a bit. Though it may feel counterintuitive, exercise improves energy levels. It's a good idea to look at other reasons why you may be feeling tired during the day, instead of always identifying a poor night of sleep as the culprit.

Belief 13 states, "I believe insomnia is essentially the result of a chemical imbalance." This simply isn't true. Research doesn't support the idea that most people with insomnia have some sort of chemical imbalance. Plus, if you agree with this statement, you probably think your insomnia is completely out of your control and that sleeping pills are the only answer. But in fact, most insomnia is actually due to a combination of behaviors and thoughts that condition the person to sleep poorly. Changing those behaviors and thoughts can help you decondition yourself and overcome your insomnia.

Belief 14 states, "I feel insomnia is ruining my ability to enjoy life and prevents me from doing what I want." This is a dysfunctional belief because insomnia itself doesn't prevent you from enjoying life and doing what you want. Each time you decide not to go out with friends, not to go to dinner with your partner, not to play outside with your children, or not to join coworkers for a get-together after work, you're making your own decision. If you believe that going out will prevent you from sleeping well that night or if you decide you just aren't up to it due to a poor night of sleep the previous night, you're allowing insomnia to take control over your decisions. In truth, you may find that you sleep better when you do the things you enjoy, and that going out with friends or family can distract you from ruminating about your sleep. Rather than turn down these opportunities, you should start to enjoy life more and observe whether it helps improve your sleep.

Belief 15 states, "Medication is probably the only solution to sleeplessness." This is certainly a dysfunctional belief, but it's one shared by many people. To a large degree, this is because the pharmaceutical companies have done such a wonderful job of advertising directly to you, the consumer. In addition, many primary care physicians don't learn enough about sleep medicine, so they aren't aware that there are better treatment options. The American Academy of Sleep Medicine recommends psychological and behavioral interventions for the treatment of both primary and secondary insomnia, due to the proven effectiveness of this approach in well-designed research trials (Morgenthaler et al. 2006). Sleeping pills are certainly not the only answer to sleeplessness.

Belief 16 states, "I avoid or cancel obligations (social, family) after a poor night's sleep." If you avoid or cancel social and family obligations due to a poor night of sleep, you're actually losing out on opportunities to help improve your sleep. It's best to try to maintain as normal a life as possible, regardless of how many hours you sleep each night. Once again, when you start canceling activities due to poor sleep, you're allowing your sleep to control your life. If you stay home or spend more time by yourself, you're more likely to dwell on your sleep problem, and that will only increase your anxiety. Make a conscious effort to enjoy life more. You don't want to miss out on social and family opportunities due to your sleep.

When Suzanne told a friend about how anxious and worried she felt, her friend suggested that she get some help. Suzanne agreed that she needed to take action in order to improve her mood and overall well-being. She went to a cognitive-behavioral therapist for a few sessions and learned some important anxiety-reducing techniques. Then she continued her progress by attending a weekly anxiety support group, along with doing exercises from a self-help workbook. She learned that her negative automatic thoughts could be controlled by coming up with more positive, alternative thoughts and by using distraction techniques and thought stopping. She also began to see how quickly she jumped to negative conclusions about situations. By allowing herself time to stop and ask the right questions, both of herself and of others, she began to realize that she could avoid a great deal of unnecessary anxiety and confusion. Although combating distorted thinking is a process that takes time, Suzanne has already noticed a reduction in her anxiety at bedtime. She no longer lies in bed worrying about all of her problems. Instead, she focuses on peaceful, calming thoughts at bedtime and sets aside time each day to work on controlling her anxiety. Not only does she feel physically and emotionally better, but her relationships are improving as well, which is making a real impact on her life.

SUMMING UP

The way you think affects your mood and your overall view of the world. By learning how to correct cognitive distortions, decrease racing thoughts, and realistically assess your fears, you'll feel better during the day, which will only benefit how you feel at night and thereby promote your sleep. It's especially important to change any dysfunctional beliefs you may have about sleep. They can keep you stuck in patterns of thinking and behaving that are ultimately counterproductive to your sleep, and your general well-being.

CHAPTER 9

Managing Daytime Stress and Maintaining a Healthy Lifestyle

Chris is a busy attorney with a stressful job. At age forty-five, he's made partner at his law firm and feels pressure from others at work to always be at the top of his game. He has four children, ages two to ten, and his school-age children attend a pricey private school. His wife stopped working years ago to look after their children, so all of the financial responsibilities in the household fall on Chris's shoulders. He doesn't mind this, because both he and his wife think it's for the best, but at times he wishes they had two incomes. Chris often works late, typically getting home around 8 or 9 p.m. He misses having dinner with his family but finds it difficult to get home any earlier. On the weekends, he tries to catch up on bills and other household duties, and to spend time with his kids. He stopped exercising years ago, as he feels he just can't find the time in his day. He drinks several cups of coffee in the morning, skips breakfast, and usually has another cup or two of coffee at lunchtime. He orders his lunch from local restaurants and tends to eat at his desk while working. Except for company functions, he and his wife don't go out much or spend time just enjoying life together. He lies in bed at night thinking about everything he has to do the next day. Chris feels stressed-out most of the time but doesn't see how he can possibly change this, and he thinks it must be part and parcel of being a high-powered attorney.

Chris's story isn't exceptional. In our fast-paced culture, many of us feel stressed on a daily basis. This epidemic of stress may in part be responsible for the current prevalence of sleep problems. Because the stress you feel during the day can affect your sleep at night, this chapter will help you learn to manage your daytime stress in a healthy way. If you incorporate stress-management skills into your daily routine, you're less likely to carry your worries into your bedtime hours. Coping skills for handling stress fall into two categories: behavioral and cognitive. Behavioral approaches include exercising, finding time to relax, eating well, and even taking a time-out when needed. Cognitive approaches include setting aside worry time and seeking support from family and friends. This chapter will help you learn how to better handle stress during the day so that it won't keep you up at night.

BEHAVIORAL TECHNIQUES

Learning to manage your daytime stress in a healthier way will probably entail changing some of your current behaviors. For example, if you typically react to stressful situations in unhealthy ways that make you feel worse in the end, then there's room for improvement in how you deal with stress. Different techniques are more effective for different people, so give all of the suggestions in this chapter a try to see which work best for you. Some of these behavioral changes may be harder to implement than others, but you owe it to yourself to give each a chance to work.

Relaxation Exercises

Incorporating relaxation exercises into your daily routine can reduce your stress and help you handle difficult situations better. For example, deep breathing exercises are an excellent way to slow down your breath rate, which increases when you're stressed-out, and to focus on feeling calm and relaxed. Next time you feel yourself becoming anxious or upset, or find yourself worrying about something, take a five-minute break to do some deep breathing. Afterward, you should feel more relaxed and better able to focus on the task at hand. This is true for all of the relaxation exercises in chapter 5. Practicing guided imagery or progressive muscle relaxation can help you feel less stressed during the day. If you work, your lunch break is a good time to practice relaxation exercises. Similarly, doing these types of exercises in the evening after a stressful day is a good way for you to clear your mind and just take ten or fifteen minutes for yourself.

Healthy Diet

Eating well can help you handle stress better. Healthy foods give you natural energy and stamina, whereas unhealthy foods can make you feel drained and fatigued. Many people cope with stress by eating, and healthy foods generally aren't at the top of the list at these times. Perhaps you grab a box of cookies, a bag of chips, or a sugary drink. Although coping with stress by eating junk food isn't uncommon, it also isn't the best idea. It can fill you up with empty calories, so that you won't be as inclined to eat nutrient-rich food, which is essential for optimal functioning of your brain and body. It can also increase your chances of gaining weight. Perhaps worst of all, eating junk food when you feel stressed is likely to backfire, as the added sugar, salt, fat, and caffeine in these foods can actually lead you to feel more physically stressed (Magee 2004).

If stress is the only reason you're eating, the best bet is to avoid eating until you're hungry. But if you are genuinely hungry, reach for a healthful snack instead. Here are some suggestions. These are better alternatives to junk food and can help refuel and reenergize your body when you need it:

- Carrot sticks and other raw vegetables with hummus, vegetable dip, or salsa

- Pita bread with hummus or eggplant dip

- Granola bar

- Raw nuts (preferably low-salt or no-salt)

- Fresh or dried fruit

- Natural peanut butter on crackers or celery sticks

- Mini whole wheat bagel with peanut butter or low-fat cream cheese

To help avoid the urge to snack altogether, start off each day the right way: with breakfast. There's a reason why so many nutrition experts consider breakfast to be the most important meal of the day: Eating breakfast kick-starts your metabolism. It also promotes stable blood sugar levels. If you haven't eaten since the night before, your body is essentially fasting, and you need to replenish your energy with healthful food. Although other meals are important as well, skipping breakfast can lead to decreased energy during the day.

For optimum health and well-being, and for steady energy throughout the day, most experts recommend eating foods that are rich in protein and complex carbohydrates, with a focus on fresh fruits and vegetables, legumes, and whole grains (Kemper and Shannon 2007). Protein-rich foods include soy, dairy, and meat, while complex carbohydrates include whole vegetables, legumes, grains, and whole grain products, such as bread, cereal, and pasta. Whole grains have a better nutritional profile than refined grains, including more fiber, and are therefore a better alternative. Because it takes longer to digest complex carbohydrates, they give you a steady stream of energy and limit the amount of sugar that is converted to fat and stored in your body. Refined carbohydrates, as found in white flour, other refined grains, and highly sweetened foods such as cake, candy, and cookies, rapidly release their sugars into the bloodstream, so they can upset your blood sugar balance and increase the chances that your body will convert these sugars to fat, particularly if you eat too much of this type of food at once.

Here are some tips for eating healthier, and thus decreasing some stress in your life.

Start with breakfast every day. Healthy starts to your day include whole-grain cereals, low-fat yogurt with fruit, or toast with a slice of cheese, an egg, or both. By eating breakfast, you'll be less likely to become overly hungry later in the day.

Eat balanced meals throughout the day. Your body needs nutrients from various sources, so try to incorporate different fruits and vegetables into your meals, along with nuts, whole grains, and protein. By eating nutritious, balanced meals, you can decrease cravings for junk food and improve your mood and energy level.

Be prepared with healthy snacks during the day. This may mean bringing along snacks when you're at work or away from home. If you have nutritious snacks available, like mixed nuts, dried or fresh fruit, carrot sticks, whole grain granola bars, yogurt, or cut-up veggies, you'll be less likely to go for cookies, chips, a candy bar, or a sugar-laden cola. Try to get rid of the junk food in your house and replace it with healthier snacks. It's okay to have a cookie now and then, of course, but if you find yourself eating junk food on a regular basis, you'll have an easier time avoiding it if you don't keep it around.

Don't skip meals. You need good nutrition in order to maintain your energy level and feel good. Some people find that eating smaller, more frequent meals helps keep their energy level more stable throughout the day. This is important for keeping your mood stable as well.

Cut out or decrease caffeine. If you're sensitive to the effects of caffeine, it would be a good idea to try decreasing your daily intake. Not only can caffeine affect your sleep at night, it can also change your mood and energy level. Because caffeine is a stimulant, when its effects wear off you may feel more sluggish than if you had skipped it in the first place. Sensitivity to caffeine is individualized, so this may or may not be the case for you. In any case, if you feel stressed during the day, grabbing a cup of coffee or other caffeinated beverage is unlikely to help, and the stimulant effect may actually make the situation worse. Instead, avoid the caffeine and find other ways to cope with stress.

Watch how much alcohol you drink. Alcohol is a depressant. Although one drink may relax you, if you already feel upset about something alcohol can make you feel worse. If you regularly turn to alcohol when you feel stressed, it's important to look at why you do this. It's not a good way to deal with stress, as it typically allows you to avoid whatever is upsetting you. Plus, it could turn into a drinking problem in the future. Find other ways to relieve stress in your life.

Leisure Activities

Having some fun can decrease your stress. Going out to dinner or the movies or inviting friends over for a get-together can help take your mind off your worries or stress and allow you to enjoy yourself. Is it difficult for you to take time to have fun? Although many people feel this way, it isn't a healthy attitude. We all deserve to have some fun, and laughing and enjoying yourself with others are great ways of reducing stress. In fact, some research suggests that humor and laughter can have beneficial effects on health, including reduced levels of stress hormones, improved of mood, reduced pain, increased creativity, improved immunity, and even reduced blood pressure (Hassed 2001). By having fun during the day, you can help yourself sleep better at night. With less worries on your mind, you'll be better able to relax at bedtime. If you aren't in the habit of doing things just for fun, you may need a little help to get started on incorporating more leisure activities into your schedule. Here's a list of a few activities many people find enjoyable, with space at the bottom for you to add more. Check off any of these activities that are fun for you, then make a commitment to do these activities more often:

_____ Going out to dinner with friends or family

_____ Going to the movies

_____ Going dancing

_____ Watching a movie at home

_____ Inviting friends or family over

_____ Going to a park

_____ Going to the beach

_____ Going to a museum

_____ Going to the theater for a concert, play, or other performance

_____ Going to a comedy club

_____ Taking a weekend vacation

_____ Going to a bookstore or the library

_____ Meeting friends at a café

_____ Playing cards or board games with friends

_____ Doing puzzles

_____ Engaging in a hobby

_____ Doing something creative, like music, art, or writing

_____ Going for a walk or a hike

_____ Going to the spa for a massage, facial, or other relaxing treatment

_____ Playing with your children

_____ Other: _____

_____ Other: _____

_____ Other: _____

_____ Other: _____

Physical Exercise

Physical exercise can be a great way to help manage daytime stress. Research has shown that vigorous physical exercise on a regular basis can improve your mood, boost your energy level, lower risk of heart disease, decrease weight problems, lessen pain, improve daytime performance, and even improve sleep (Kemper and Shannon 2007; Leppämäki et al. 2004). In addition to all of these great reasons for exercising, it can also help calm your mind. As mentioned in chapter 8, you may tend to worry or ruminate during monotonous forms of exercise, like swimming or jogging. So with these types of exercise, it's especially important to really focus on what you're doing. If you're swimming, think about your strokes, your breathing, and how good the water feels. If you go for a run, focus on your stride and keeping an even pace. Listening to music while you exercise can also help keep your mind off your worries. Sing along if you want, or just enjoy your favorite tunes. By focusing on what you're doing and keeping yourself free of worries and anxiety while exercising, you can take an important step in managing your daytime stress.

Although exercising every day is optimal in terms of health, you may have trouble finding the time for this. Plus, if you've been mostly inactive, it's important to start slowly. As you begin your exercise program, try to exercise at least two times per week. Schedule some time to exercise and stick with it. Once you start noticing the benefits of regular physical exercise, you're likely to want to do it more and more often. In addition, finding activities that you enjoy and that work in your schedule is important to the success of your exercise program. Of course, if you have any serious medical conditions or are worried about exercising due to health concerns, you should consult with your doctor first before beginning an exercise program.

SPICE UP YOUR EXERCISE ROUTINE

Alternating your activities can be a great way to keep your exercise program fresh and decrease your chances of getting bored or not sticking with it. Here's an example: If you plan to exercise three times a week, during the first week you could walk at a fast pace two times per week and attend a class on another day. During the second week, you could go for a bicycle ride one day, hop on a treadmill another day, and take a brisk walk the third day.

Going to a group exercise class can be a fun and engaging way to exercise more. From step aerobics and kick boxing to body sculpting classes to yoga and Pilates, there is a huge variety of options from which to choose, so you're bound to find something that works for you. If high-impact activities are difficult or painful for you, water aerobics, low-impact aerobics, yoga, and Pilates may be easier on your body. If you think the typical gym environment isn't for you, be aware that there are plenty of classes oriented to different types of people, including seniors and pregnant women. Another advantage of classes is that being with other people and following a teacher's instructions may encourage you to challenge yourself more than you would on your own.

If you have children, get them involved in your exercise routine as well. You can go jogging while little ones ride their bikes alongside, or the entire family can go biking together. If you take your kids to a playground, you can run and climb with them, rather than simply sitting on a park bench and watching. If your children are older, why not go for a walk together before or after dinner? It's a nice way to spend time together and catch up on events of the day while also doing something positive for your health.

Finding an exercise buddy can be a great way to help you stick with an exercise program. Just by agreeing to walk with a friend, for example, you're making a commitment to improve your health. Plus, you have someone else who is counting on you to exercise. This can be the best type of motivation, because not only will you be exercising, you'll also be connecting with a friend while you do it. Try going for a bike ride or taking a brisk walk with a friend.

OPTIMAL TIMES TO EXERCISE

Keep in mind that in order to improve your sleep and not worsen it, the timing of your exercise is important. As mentioned in chapter 4, exercising about four to five hours before bedtime is ideal. If you can't exercise then, exercise in the morning or even during your lunch break. If your office is near your home, how about riding your bike to work? Or perhaps you work near a gym, where you can exercise for thirty minutes and still be back at your office on time. Other options include taking a walk at lunchtime—as long as you still leave yourself enough time to eat a nutritious lunch. By exercising in the morning or four to five hours before bedtime, you'll help manage your daytime stress and improve your nighttime sleep at the same time.

Documenting Your Exercise Program

To ensure your success in following your exercise program, you'll need to make a commitment to doing so. After you've considered all of the information above and given some thought to what types of exercise you'd most enjoy doing, use the following worksheet to schedule what you intend to do, and then stick to it. You may want to make copies so you'll always have a blank form to use as you change your exercise program in the future.

Week of (dates):	Type of Exercise	Time of Day
Monday		
Tuesday		
Wednesday		
Thursday		
Friday		
Saturday		
Sunday		

Taking a Time-Out

Time-outs work for children, so why not try one yourself? Taking a time-out can be a helpful way to regain your focus, calm down, and put things in perspective when you're feeling stressed-out or upset. There is a reason time-outs are used when children get upset or throw a fit: it works. You may not be throwing a fit, but you can still benefit from taking yourself out of a stressful situation for a few minutes in order to think more clearly. Do you remember your parents or grandparents telling you to count to ten when you got upset? It's the same concept. When you feel stressed-out, taking a five- or ten-minute time-out can feel like a lifesaver. Here are some guidelines for taking an effective time-out:

1. Physically separate yourself from the environment that's causing the stress. For example, this may mean excusing yourself from others and going into another room or taking a short walk outside.

2. Try to slow down your breathing and heart rate. Take a few deep breaths or use any of the breathing exercises in chapter 5 to help calm you down and decrease the stress and anxiety you feel.

3. Don't rush back into the stressful situation. Take at least five to ten minutes to calm yourself down and think about the situation.

4. If you return to the stressful situation after your time-out, try to remain calm. There's no point in upsetting yourself again. That will only take a greater toll on your mind and body.

There are numerous benefits to taking a time-out when you feel stressed. It can help you collect your thoughts without being bothered or interrupted by others. It can give you time to figure out a solution to the problem, even if it's only a short-term fix. While in a time-out, you can take a few deep breaths and calm yourself down so you feel better physically and mentally. Physical separation from an upsetting situation can be important during stressful times. Plus, it can give you a chance to put things in perspective. Is this situation worth getting so upset over? Is it taking a greater toll on your well-being than is warranted?

Stepping aside from a stressful situation and calming yourself increases the chance that you'll respond in a rational, more thoughtful way. When you react to stressful situations impulsively, you can end up regretting your words and actions later. It's much better to take a time-out when needed than to react immediately and later be further upset by your response. This is an important lesson to learn. Not only will it improve the way you handle stress, it will also improve your relationships with other people.

COGNITIVE TECHNIQUES

The stress management skills discussed so far have been focused on behavioral approaches to leading a healthier, less stressful life. Relaxation exercises, a healthy diet, engaging in fun leisure activities, getting enough exercise, and knowing when to take a time-out are all part of a positive and healthy lifestyle. You can also use cognitive techniques to reduce your daytime stress. Some of these were covered in the previous chapter, on controlling anxiety and irrational thoughts. Hopefully you're continuing to work on correcting cognitive distortions and racing thoughts. Because doing so involves changing long-term habitual thought patterns, it may take some time. Meanwhile, here are some simple cognitive strategies that will help you manage your daytime stress.

Worry Time

One way to help decrease a tendency to focus on anxious thoughts while you're lying in bed at night is to manage some of your worries during the day. Try setting aside a time each day to write down some of your biggest worries. By writing down these thoughts during the day, you can start to address what's bothering you. Try to make time to do this every day. It can be whenever is convenient for you as long as it isn't too late at night, because you don't want these worries to be on your mind when you get into bed. Simply write down what your worry is and how you're handling it or how you plan to handle it. Then, if the same worry pops into your head while you're lying in bed at night, you can remind yourself that you already addressed it during your designated worry time and that you've already come up with a solution. Assure your mind that you've dealt with that worry and it need not disturb your sleep anymore.

Although this technique may seem like a simple or even silly thing to do, it really can make a difference. If you find yourself worrying a lot at night, this technique will be especially helpful for you. If you try it for a couple of weeks and your sleep doesn't improve, then daytime worries probably aren't causing your sleep problem, so you can move on to other approaches that work better for you.

Documenting Your Worries

You can write your worries in any format that works for you: in a notebook, on index cards with one worry on each card, or even in a journal reserved just for your worries. But if you'd like a little help getting started, here's a worry-time worksheet. The main thing is to write down whatever you find yourself worrying about, and then write down what you're doing to deal with the situation, or what you plan to do about it.

What are your worries or concerns? Be specific; for example, are they financial problems, marital or relationship conflicts, problems with your children, work-related issues, your health, or something else?

_____

_____

_____

_____

_____

_____

_____

What are you doing to handle these concerns? Again, be specific; for example, are you saving more money, communicating more and working on your relationship with your spouse or partner, reaching out to your children, talking with your boss or coworkers more, exercising and eating right, or something else? What's your solution?

_____

_____

_____

_____

_____

_____

_____

By taking time each day to write down a few of your worries and how you're addressing them, you can decrease your overall stress. The next time one of these worries enters your mind, you can remind yourself that you're already aware of it and taking care of it. You've written down a solution of how to handle the worry.

Support From Family and Friends

Do you tend to keep things bottled up inside? Perhaps you avoid telling family or friends about your problems or worries because you think they won't really care or just don't want to hear about it. Or maybe you think you'll be a burden to others if you tell them what's really going on in your life. Alternatively, you may feel that it's best to keep your problems to yourself because telling others is a sign of weakness.

These types of feelings and fears are quite common. Many people don't reach out to others because they're scared of the reaction they'll receive, or because they don't want to "blow their cover" and let on that not everything is perfect and peachy in their lives. But the reality is that everyone has problems, and it can be helpful to talk with family and friends about what's bothering you. Plus, it can actually improve your relationships with others, because you'll be more honest about how you're feeling and what you're experiencing each day.

You may wonder how reaching out to others can help you manage your daytime stress. Think of the last time you became very stressed-out at work or at home. Did you tell anyone about it, or did you simply hold your frustrations inside? If you told someone, then you already know the benefits of sharing your feelings with others. Not only are you able to let go of some of your frustration, and the stress that goes along with it, you may also get valuable feedback from others. When you're under a lot of stress and are focused on that stress, it may be difficult to have a good perspective on the world around you. By talking with others about the stress or worries in your life, you can hear what someone else thinks about it. Sometimes that alone can be enough to remind you of what's really important.

One day at work, Chris felt a pain in his arm and started having trouble breathing. A coworker rushed him to the hospital, where he was told that he was about to have a heart attack and was lucky that he'd arrived to the ER when he did. This shocked Chris. What was the point of all of his hard work if he died at age forty-five from a heart attack? After talking with his doctor and his wife, Chris decided that he had to slow down and decrease his stress for his own health and well-being. The idea of change didn't come easy for Chris, who was used to a fast-paced life. He started with small steps, like drinking less coffee and having a healthy breakfast with his family. Not only did his children love having breakfast with their dad, but Chris also found the time to be very fulfilling. Chris also decided to bring a healthy lunch to work with him, rather than always ordering food from restaurants, and he cut out his lunchtime coffee. As he took these small steps, he began to feel the difference, both physically and mentally, and this helped motivate him to make bigger changes.

The hardest change for Chris was deciding that he wouldn't ever stay at work past 6 p.m. The first few days he felt a little guilty about it, but then he noticed that he wasn't the only person at the office leaving at that time and realized that he had been too consumed with his work before. Seeing how out of balance his life was, he also realized that he needed to take some time out on a regular basis to have fun with family and friends. Since there's a gym in Chris's office building, he decided to go to the gym after work for thirty minutes each day. This still put him home before 7 p.m., allowing him to have dinner with his family each evening. Chris's wife decided to take a part-time job that she could do from home, so Chris's worries about finances decreased.

Upon the recommendation of his doctor, Chris also attended a series of stress management workshops at his local hospital and learned different ways to cope with and manage stress. For example, he started talking with his wife and friends about his worries, and this seemed to work well for him. Six months after nearly suffering a heart attack, Chris was gratified and relieved when his doctor said that his health was much better and to keep up the good work.

SUMMING UP

Daytime stress that isn't managed well can keep you up at night. For that reason, it's important to learn a wide variety of stress-management techniques and determine which work best for you. Different techniques may be more effective depending on the type of stress you face. So one day you may find it helpful to play golf to get some exercise, another day you may need a time-out at work when you're confronted with a frustrating situation, and on another day you may want to treat yourself to a back massage. The key is to be aware of what works for you in different situations, and to motivate yourself by remembering that decreasing stress in your life can improve your physical and emotional health.

CHAPTER 10

Preventing Relapse

Jill is a twenty-eight-year-old nurse who experienced insomnia off and on in her early twenties. She always thought her problem was due to working rotating shifts, but for the past few years she's only worked the day shift. About a year ago, she had a bad bout of insomnia. At that time, she had just broken up with her fiancé and was feeling quite depressed. She attended therapy for her depression, but once her symptoms of depression lifted, her sleep problems remained. For that reason, she consulted with a sleep specialist who treated her with cognitive behavioral techniques. By changing her sleep hygiene, keeping a sleep log, and utilizing both stimulus control and sleep restriction, she was back to sleeping well again after a few weeks. She was able to handle an occasional bad night of sleep by not worrying too much about it and maintaining what she'd learned.

For about six months, she continued to get good sleep almost every night, but all of that changed a few months ago when she started dating someone new. Her sleep schedule became more erratic, and her sleep hygiene started to deteriorate. Her boyfriend liked to watch TV in bed, which kept her awake, and she found herself struggling with how to handle it. Since she wasn't getting to sleep until later at night, she felt so exhausted during the day that she started having a couple of cups of coffee in the afternoon. At first these changes didn't seem to affect her sleep, but then one night she noticed herself staring at the clock and worrying about work, her relationship, and everything else in her life. With her boyfriend sleeping next to her, she was embarrassed to get up out of bed after fifteen or twenty minutes of sleeplessness like she'd learned, so she laid in bed counting the minutes for what seemed like an eternity. She got out of bed the next morning more anxious than ever, convinced that she was destined to be plagued by insomnia.

Now that you've come this far in the sleep program, you should be sleeping much better, as Jill was after working with a sleep specialist. You've learned how your thoughts and behaviors affect your sleep, and you've put that information to work by practicing good sleep hygiene, following the stimulus control and sleep restriction guidelines, and taking control of anxiety both during the day and at night. There's just one step remaining: making sure that you continue to sleep well. One of the most important strategies in this regard is not to let an occasional bad night convince you that you're back on the road to an ongoing sleep problem. Quite the contrary—everyone experiences a poor night of sleep once in a while. Don't become frustrated if it happens to you and you fall into the same trap as Jill, thinking you have no control over the situation. Instead, focus on how you can maintain good sleeping patterns through positive thoughts and behaviors.

KEEP UP THE GOOD WORK

Even when you're sleeping better, it's important to maintain good sleep hygiene. Since you've had sleep problems in the past, you don't want to increase your chances of having them occur again. For example, restricting the amount of caffeine you consume after 12 noon is always a good idea, because caffeine can remain in your body for long periods of time. Similarly, exercising four to five hours before bedtime (or earlier in the day), instead of later in the evening, is important because you don't want to increase your body temperature, which makes it difficult to fall asleep.

Maintaining good sleep hygiene also means remembering not to do activities in bed that are stimulating or promote wakefulness. Since your bed should be reserved for sleep and sex only, remember to talk on the phone or check your e-mail in another room. The same goes for watching TV or reading in bed. Similarly, continue to cover your clock so you aren't tempted to watch the clock when you have a more restless night than usual. Remember, clock watching only exacerbates anxiety related to sleep. Likewise, continue to avoid bright light in the evenings so your circadian rhythm isn't disrupted. By establishing and maintaining good sleep hygiene, you will decrease your chances of having another bout of insomnia in the future.

Knowing what affects your sleep will help you maintain good sleep hygiene and prevent new episodes of insomnia. By keeping a sleep log, as described in chapter 6, you've probably learned a great deal about the factors that affect your sleep. Perhaps you noticed that having a heavy or spicy meal for dinner disrupted your sleep, or that a midafternoon cappuccino kept you up at night. Similarly, you may have noticed that your sleep is more disrupted after a few drinks, or that the timing of exercise can impact your sleep. To maintain your gains, you need to stay aware of these factors so that they don't cause sleep problems in the future.

Hopefully you've made changes in your life to minimize the effect these factors have on your sleep. If you have, you should be proud of yourself. Changing your behavior and habits is hard work, and changing your thinking patterns may be even harder! Doing so takes willpower and perseverance. Having come so far in improving your sleep, it's important to continue to cultivate the positive new habits you've developed as you've worked through this book. Once you're sleeping better, you may be tempted to stop using the various techniques you've learned in this book. However, it's best to maintain these sleep-promoting lifestyle changes. You need to continue to find time to connect with family and friends, do relaxation exercises, maintain a healthy diet, get enough exercise, have fun, and more. In other words, you need to continue to work for that "perfect balance" in your life. Likewise, continue to work toward managing daily stress without becoming too upset or anxious, and maintaining a positive attitude regarding your sleep. By keeping up the good work you've done so far, you can continue to sleep well into the future.

WAYS TO HANDLE AN OCCASIONAL BAD NIGHT

To help you deal with an occasional poor night of sleep, keep in mind that it's quite common to have difficulty sleeping on occasion, and it doesn't mean that you're headed down the path toward more sleepless nights. Try to figure out what caused the problem. Were you worried about something at work? Did you have a conflict with your spouse or significant other, or with other family members? Were financial problems on your mind? Were you excited about something happening the next day, like a party or a trip? Did you have a heavy meal that caused indigestion, or did you drink too much alcohol while out with friends?

Situations like these, and many other factors, can cause temporary insomnia for just a night or two. The key is to not let it turn into a chronic problem again. The best way to do that is not to make too big a deal out of it, and to maintain good sleep habits. By not overreacting to an occasional bad night's sleep, you take a realistic, not distorted, view of the situation. You don't feed your anxiety about not sleeping, which fuels a vicious cycle that can lead to chronic sleep problems.

Resisting the Sleeping Pill Trap

If you have an occasional bad night of sleep, don't give in to the temptation to take a sleeping pill. This just leads to psychological dependence—the idea that you lack the ability to sleep well without medications. By now, you should know this isn't the case. And if you do give in and take sleep medications and continue taking them, your body will become dependent on them, which will create even worse insomnia once you stop taking the medication. As you've worked through this book, you've learned how to overcome insomnia on your own, without sleeping pills, so you really don't need them.

Don't Let Your Thoughts Run Away with Your Sleep

An occasional bad night of sleep is just that: an *occasional* bad night of sleep. Don't let yourself believe it means anything more than that. Throughout this sleep program, you've seen how your thoughts can affect your sleep. If you continue to have negative thoughts or dysfunctional beliefs about your sleep, go back to chapter 8 and address those thoughts and beliefs again. When you've thought a certain way for a long time, you may automatically go back to thinking that way again, particularly in times of stress. That's why it's so important to keep practicing the new cognitive techniques you've learned, so that your new, positive, sleep-promoting and anxiety-reducing thoughts will become habits that can replace thoughts and beliefs that might get in the way of sleeping well.

Keep Practicing What You've Learned

Perhaps by now you sense a theme. The key to maintaining good sleep is to keep practicing what you've learned in this book: observing good sleep hygiene, practicing relaxation exercises, following the guidelines for stimulus control and sleep restriction (if need be), controlling anxiety and correcting cognitive distortions, and managing daytime stress. Continue to incorporate all of these practices into your life. It's especially important to keep the principles of stimulus control in mind. For example, if you're unable to sleep for fifteen or twenty minutes, you need to get out of bed, go into another room, and do something boring or relaxing until you feel sleepy. Remember to do this even if you just have an occasional bad night of sleep, because you don't want to once again build up an association between your bed and frustration or negative thoughts—especially after you've worked so hard to undo those associations. By continuing to practice everything you've learned, you can decrease your chances of having a sleep problem in the future.

TAKING CARE OF UNDERLYING DEPRESSION OR ANXIETY

As discussed in chapter 2, some people with sleep problems also have depression or anxiety that is separate from their insomnia. Although this book can still help anyone sleep better, if you have depression or anxiety, you may need help specific to those issues. It's important that you get the help that you need from a qualified mental health professional, such as a psychologist or psychiatrist. Start by talking to your primary care physician about your symptoms and asking for advice on where to find help. If you resist the idea of getting help, remember this: Because both depression and anxiety can have a negative impact on sleep, you'll be at increased risk of insomnia in the future if either problem remains untreated.

If Your Sleep Is Better but You Still Feel Down in the Dumps

If you're sleeping better after using the approaches described in this book but you still feel depressed, you probably have a mood disorder and would benefit from treatment for depression. Sometimes people don't realize they have a separate mood disorder until after their insomnia has improved. If depression is an issue for you, perhaps you always thought it was related to your insomnia. For many people it is. But for others, depression remains after a sleep problem has been resolved. Feeling depressed can be very distressing and have a significant negative impact on your life, making you feel helpless or hopeless and leading you to avoid social situations. But you don't need to continue suffering. There are many effective treatments for depression.

If you're scared to admit that you may be depressed, you aren't alone. It's hard to face the facts of depression. You may feel that it's something you should be able to get over on your own, without help from anyone else. After all, you've always managed to solve your own problems. Why should depression be any different? Unfortunately, trying to deal with depression by yourself can be a very difficult task. Symptoms of depression include sadness, lack of interest in activities, fatigue or loss of energy, feelings of worthlessness or excessive guilt, decreased attention and concentration, weight changes, and thoughts of suicide. Not only are these symptoms very distressing, many of them make it difficult for you to overcome depression on your own. Don't be nervous or hesitant about asking others for help. It's an important thing to be able to do, and it actually shows real strength of character.

Many resources are available that can help you overcome depression. First of all, it's a good idea to tell your family practitioner or primary care physician about how you've been feeling. Most doctors see people with depression every day and may have good local referrals for you. Options for treatment include individual psychotherapy (particularly cognitive behavioral therapy), support groups, and antidepressant medications. It's important not to ignore the symptoms because they affect how you feel every day and diminish your overall quality of life. Find the help you need so that you can start feeling better and enjoying life again.

If You Continue to Worry About Many Things Unrelated to Sleep

If you find yourself struggling with anxiety, such as constant worries, difficulty relaxing, and ruminating over problems throughout the day, then your anxiety is taking quite a toll on your life. If these worries don't relate to your sleep problem, you have a problem with anxiety that's separate from your insomnia. As you've worked through this book, you've learned various techniques to help deal with your anxiety. Continue to practice the exercises in chapter 8, which can help you manage and control your anxiety by allowing you to see things in a different way. If you feel like you need additional help, various options are available to you.

As with depression, cognitive behavioral therapy is very effective for anxiety. Some people also benefit from antianxiety medications depending on the severity of their anxiety. However, since you've experienced sleep problems, it's a good idea for you to avoid taking benzodiazepines for anxiety, as you might be tempted to use them for sleep. If your doctor recommends that you take an antianxiety medication and you want to give it a try, discuss this concern with your doctor. Other medications, such as buspirone (BuSpar) and certain SSRI antidepressants approved by the FDA for anxiety, carry less potential for dependency. Whether you decide to treat your anxiety through pharmacological or nonpharmacological methods is an important decision that only you can make. But if your anxiety is bothering you during the day, seeking some sort of help for this problem should be a high priority, as it takes a toll on your life.

If you've lived with anxiety for many years, you may have trouble remembering a time when you didn't experience the constant worries in your life. Perhaps you aren't aware of how much anxiety negatively impacts you on a day-to-day basis. It can make you less likely to enjoy activities, due to racing thoughts and worries. It can make it hard for you to really relax, because you tend to feel keyed up or nervous much of the time. It can also affect your social relationships. You may skip going out with people due to fears, preoccupations, or worries, or people may pick up on your anxiety and feel uncomfortable around you. In either case, you're likely to become more socially isolated. Anxiety can also affect your physical health; for example, you may experience ulcers, frequent headaches, back or shoulder pain, or many other symptoms.

Cognitive behavioral treatment for anxiety is similar to the approaches described in chapter 8. It involves changing negative, irrational thoughts and fears to more positive, rational thoughts and addressing any dysfunctional beliefs that are causing significant anxiety. In other words, if the way you think is making your anxiety worse, learning to think in different ways will decrease your anxiety and help you start feeling better overall. Altering your behaviors is also an important part of overcoming anxiety. By practicing relaxation exercises, you can learn to stop anxiety that's building up inside of you before it becomes unmanageable. You can also learn what tends to trigger your anxiety and then come up with better ways to cope with those situations. Once you start feeling more comfortable in anxiety-provoking situations, you'll feel better overall. With fewer worries, irrational thoughts, and fears, you can enjoy life more and not feel overwhelmed by your anxiety.

> *Jill's story is a common one. Believing that she was no longer susceptible to insomnia, she stopped practicing good sleep hygiene and other techniques she'd learned. As she fell back into her old habits, and because of new circumstances in her life, she found she wasn't immune to sleeplessness. Fortunately, after a few sleepless nights Jill was frustrated enough that she decided to take control of the situation rather than start down the path of chronic insomnia again. Right away, she stopped having caffeine in the afternoons and stuck with just one cup of coffee in the morning. Talking with her boyfriend was harder. Although she'd never discussed her sleep problem with anyone other than her doctor before, she explained her history to her boyfriend. He hadn't realized that she was having trouble sleeping, or that he was contributing to the problem, and he immediately agreed to help her make some needed changes. They stopped watching TV in bed in the evening and instead watched it in the living room. They also decided that setting a regular bedtime was an important step in helping Jill get back on track.*
>
> *Jill explained stimulus control to her boyfriend and told him that if she found herself lying in bed awake for too long, she needed to get up, and that he shouldn't worry or wonder about her when she did this. Just talking about the situation with her boyfriend seemed to help decrease her anxiety, and his supportive response helped ease many of her concerns about the relationship. Over the next month, Jill had a few more bad nights, but she realized that these were just temporary, and perhaps part of getting used to a new person and new routines in her life. As she continued to maintain her good sleep hygiene and adjust to her new situation, she started sleeping well again most every night.*

SUMMING UP

Everyone has an occasional bad night of sleep. If you keep that in mind and don't make too much out of it, you can save yourself a lot of anxiety and unnecessary frustration. If you've found that you have depression or anxiety that seems to be unrelated to your insomnia, you need to seek help for these symptoms. There's no reason why you should continue to suffer with untreated depression or anxiety, or their consequences, so don't delay any longer in getting the help you need.

Restful, restorative sleep is so important for your health and overall well-being. The time and energy you devote to practicing the techniques in this book will amply reward you with better sleep, and a better quality of life. The next two chapters will address issues that may not apply to you: parasomnias and special considerations for women in regard to sleep. If neither is relevant to you, then perhaps your reading will end here. If so, I wish you many years of sleeping well and awakening refreshed and renewed.

CHAPTER 11

Parasomnias

Parasomnias are behaviors that intrude into sleep, occur during transitions from one sleep stage to another, or occur during the transitions between sleep and waking (Rothenberg 2000). Generally considered to be undesirable at best, these behaviors either occur during sleep or are made worse by sleep (Kuhn 2001). In this chapter, I'll describe the more common parasomnias: sleepwalking, sleep terrors, confusional arousals, sleep-related eating disorder, REM sleep behavior disorder, and nightmare disorder. If the checklist in chapter 2 indicated that you may have a parasomnia, be sure to read the related section in this chapter.

SLEEPWALKING

According to the *International Classification of Sleep Disorders, somnambulism,* or sleepwalking, is a series of complex behaviors that typically begin during arousals from slow-wave sleep and result in "walking around with an altered state of consciousness and impaired judgment" (AASM 2005, 142). Because it usually occurs during slow-wave sleep, it's often seen in the first third or half of the sleep period. (You may recall from chapter 1 that most slow-wave sleep, or stage N3 sleep, occurs in the first half of the night, whereas most REM sleep occurs in the second half of the night.) Sleepwalking is thought to be a disorder of arousal because it occurs during an incomplete transition from deep sleep to wakefulness (Rothenberg 2000). Brain waves during sleepwalking indicate slow-wave sleep, but the behaviors that occur are usually associated with being awake.

Sleepwalking is quite common in childhood, with the prevalence being as high as 17 percent between ages eight and twelve (AASM 2005). The numbers drop significantly in later childhood and beyond. If you sleepwalk, you should take various precautions take to ensure a safe sleeping environment. Make sure that all windows are securely locked or blocked, and cover or remove any sharp objects. Put pillows on the floor around your bed to decrease the chance of hurting yourself during the night.

Ask everyone you live with to help you by picking up objects from the floor so you don't trip while sleepwalking. Put locks on doors to the outside up high so that you can't easily reach them and leave your house.

You can decrease the likelihood that you'll sleepwalk by not depriving yourself of sleep. When you don't get enough sleep for several nights in a row, you may experience *delta rebound*, or *slow-wave rebound*, meaning you'll have more slow-wave sleep on an upcoming night. Since sleepwalking usually occurs during slow-wave sleep, this increases your chance of sleepwalking. Besides sleep loss, other factors that can increase the chances of sleepwalking include hyperthyroidism, head injury, encephalitis, migraines, stroke, obstructive sleep apnea, and other forms of sleep-disordered breathing (AASM 2005).

One tactic that helps some people decrease sleepwalking is playing soft music or using a white noise machine while sleeping. This decreases your slow-wave sleep, so it can reduce your chance of sleepwalking. Keeping a night-light on has a similar effect. These strategies can be particularly useful if your sleepwalking is quite disruptive or if you're away from home and are nervous about sleepwalking in an unfamiliar environment. It's also important to note that certain sleep medications, such as Ambien (zolpidem), Lunesta (eszopiclone), and Sonata (zaleplon), can cause increased sleepwalking and other unusual behaviors like eating, cooking, or even driving while sleeping. Lithium carbonate, certain antipsychotic medications, and some anticholinergic medications may also increase the chances of sleepwalking (AASM 2005).

SLEEP TERRORS

Sleep terrors, also known as night terrors, are similar to sleepwalking in that they tend to start during the slow-wave period of sleep in the first third to half of the night. (You may recall from chapter 1 that most slow-wave, or stage N3 sleep, occurs in the first half of the sleep period, whereas most REM sleep occurs in the second half of the night.) An episode, which usually lasts between thirty seconds and three minutes, consists of what appears to be a state of terror, with screaming, increased heart rate, rapid breathing, dilated pupils, and movement (Broughton 1999). It's usually quite difficult to console or pacify someone who has just experienced a sleep terror. People who are awakened during a sleep terror are usually confused and disoriented and seldom remember that the episode occurred (AASM 2005). They may, however, remember frightening images or fragments of scary dreams. It is often family members or roommates who describe what happened during the episode.

As with sleepwalking, sleep terrors are more common in children, and reassurance from a parent is usually helpful. For most children, sleep terrors tend to go away on their own by adolescence. However, adults can also have sleep terrors. As with sleepwalking, slow-wave sleep rebound after sleep deprivation can exacerbate sleep terrors, so try not to have too many nights of short sleep in a row. Stress can also cause more sleep terrors, so stress reduction and stress management are helpful. Relaxation exercises, deep breathing, and psychotherapy can be helpful as well. For severe sleep terrors that are very disruptive, it may be worthwhile to consider medication. Diazepam (Valium), clonazepam (Klonopin), and certain tricyclic antidepressants can be effective for decreasing the number of episodes (Broughton 1999). However, they can also increase clumsiness and confusion, which can lead to injury. Due to the possibility of moving and walking around during an episode, it's wise to take the safety precautions mentioned for sleepwalking if you have sleep terrors.

CONFUSIONAL AROUSALS

Also called "nocturnal sleep drunkenness," confusional arousals are episodes of considerable confusion during and after arousal from sleep that don't involve sleepwalking or sleep terrors (Broughton 1999). During an episode, behavior may be inappropriate, thinking is slower and confused, and the person may not be oriented to the time or place. Because the person is only partially awake, their thinking may be unclear and illogical. Like sleepwalking and sleep terrors, confusional arousals usually occur during slow-wave sleep and the episode typically isn't remembered upon awakening in the morning.

Sedative-hypnotics, central nervous system depressants, fever, and sleep deprivation can all increase the chances of experiencing a confusional arousal, which can last from a few minutes to several hours. While about 17 percent of children have confusional arousals, only 3 to 4 percent of people age fifteen years and older have them (AASM 2005). In children they tend to be quite benign and go away with time, but in adults they can be more problematic and long-term. In adults, the risks of self-injury or injuring others during an episode are increased, performance at school or work may suffer, and chances of getting into a motor vehicle accident may also be higher if the person attempts to drive during an episode. If you've had confusional arousal episodes in the past, make sure that you wait a sufficient amount of time after awakening before engaging in any potentially dangerous activities, and ask family and friends to be aware of whether you might be experiencing an episode and to help keep you safe if they think this is the case.

Stress management may be helpful in the treatment of confusional arousals. As with other parasomnias, it's important to get enough sleep on a nightly basis, as sleep loss and subsequent slow-wave sleep rebound, can worsen episodes. Other factors that can increase the likelihood of confusional arousals include drinking alcohol, drug abuse, forced awakenings, working rotating or night shifts, and certain sleep disorders such as obstructive sleep apnea and periodic limb movement disorder (AASM 2005). Minimizing all of these factors will be very helpful in decreasing the likelihood of episodes. It's also a good idea to examine whether any of your medications could be making the problem worse. And as always, it's important to maintain good sleep hygiene.

SLEEP-RELATED EATING DISORDER

Sleep-related eating disorder occurs when you eat during your sleep. The level of consciousness during sleep-related eating disorder ranges from "virtual unconsciousness to various levels of partial consciousness" (AASM 2005, 174). In other words, when you wake up the next morning, you may have no recall of an eating episode or you may have significant recall. The eating episodes are involuntary, and odd combinations of food or inedible substances are often consumed. Injuries can occur if the person uses the stove or leaves the stove or oven on. Daytime consequences can also be severe, such as weight gain and difficulty managing high cholesterol or diabetes.

It's unclear what causes sleep related eating disorder, but it's often associated with sleepwalking, restless legs syndrome, periodic limb movement disorder, obstructive sleep apnea, and circadian rhythm disorders (Najjar 2007; AASM 2005). Similarly, people with daytime eating disorders may experience sleep-related eating disorder. In addition, sleep-related eating disorder sometimes occurs in people who are dieting or otherwise restricting their food intake during the day. Over the past few years, some research has shown that taking Ambien (zolpidem) can actually cause episodes of sleep-related eating disorder (Najjar 2007). This may be particularly true if you have an underlying sleep disorder that causes arousals, such as restless legs syndrome, periodic limb movement disorder, or obstructive sleep apnea (Morgenthaler and Silber 2002). This possible side effect—sleep-related eating disorder—is now listed with other side effects on Ambien's packaging. Episodes of sleep-related eating have also been noted with Halcion (triazolam), lithium carbonate, and certain anticholinergic medications (AASM 2005).

Some options for treatment include decreasing the chances of sleep-related eating episodes by locking kitchen cupboards and the refrigerator and putting safety latches or devices on ovens and stoves—all of which are also important for safety. When it's more difficult to perform the elaborate behaviors involved in eating and cooking during sleep, the person is more likely to either wake up during the episode or return to bed without eating.

As with sleep terrors, psychotherapy can be helpful for sleep-related eating disorder by teaching the person how to reduce or deal with stress and how to manage daytime eating behaviors. Those who also have an eating disorder should seek professional help from a specialist in this field, since the consequences of untreated eating disorders such as bulimia or anorexia can be deadly.

REM SLEEP BEHAVIOR DISORDER

Whereas the parasomnias discussed above tend to emerge from delta or slow-wave sleep, REM sleep behavior disorder (RBD) occurs during REM sleep. Part of normal REM sleep is to have muscle atonia, which is essentially paralysis. This keeps you from acting out your dreams. With RBD, people experience episodes of intense motor activity while dreaming, acting out their dreams as they occur. Often the dreams are quite violent in nature, so the movements can be explosive and involve sudden jerking, punching, kicking, jumping or diving out of bed, or crashing into furniture or walls (Broughton 1999). As a result, injuries to the sleeper or others are quite common during RBD episodes. People with RBD frequently have vivid recollection of their dreams and describe fighting or trying to escape danger.

RBD is more common in men age sixty or older, but it can affect anyone. Although a variety of neurological disorders are present in about one-third to one-half of people with RBD, the other cases are idiopathic, meaning there's no known cause. In about 50 percent of people with RBD, a central nervous system disorder such as narcolepsy, cerebrovascular disorder, or a neurodegenerative disease is present (Schenck and Mahowald 2003). In all people with RBD, however, it's likely that there is a dysfunction in the brain stem area that usually suppresses muscle tone and activity during REM sleep (Broughton 1999). Research indicates that RBD may be a precursor to developing Parkinson's disease at a later age (Berg 2008). Because the causes and treatment are different, it's important to accurately diagnose RBD and differentiate it from other disorders, like common nightmares, sleep terrors, seizures, post-traumatic stress disorder, and delirium. The best way to obtain an accurate diagnosis is with an overnight sleep study in an accredited sleep lab.

The typical treatment for RBD is medication, with clonazepam (Klonopin) appearing to be the most effective. Desipramine (Norpramin) has also been used to treat RBD. As with the parasomnias discussed above, it's very important to make the sleeping environment as safe as possible, removing all sharp objects, putting pillows on the floor next to the bed, and eliminating obstacles that could cause the person to fall or be injured during an episode. If you experience episodes of acting out your dreams, find a sleep specialist in your area who can accurately diagnosis whether you have RBD and treat you if necessary.

NIGHTMARE DISORDER

Nightmares are dreams that are frightening in nature and tend to cause you to wake up. They usually occur in the latter half of the sleep period, when REM sleep, and therefore dreaming, is more prevalent. Unlike a sleep terror, where the person may not recall any dream content or may just recall a few images, people tend to remember the dream images from nightmares in significant detail, and the content of the images is increasingly scary as the nightmare progresses (Broughton 1999). You may wake up feeling anxious, upset, scared, angry, and even embarrassed by the content of a nightmare.

While everyone has occasional nightmares, nightmare disorder involves having frequent nightmares that often cause "awakenings from sleep with recall of intensely disturbing dream mentation, usually involving fear or anxiety, but also anger, sadness, disgust, and other dysphoric emotions (AASM 2005, 156). In other words, there is a heightened emotional response upon awakening, and the content of the dream is remembered. Unlike sleep terrors, where people are confused if they're awakened during an episode, when you are awakened after having a nightmare you'll usually be fully alert and oriented and know that you just had a very bad dream. Those with nightmare disorder find it difficult to fall back asleep after having an episode, and their nightmares tend to occur in the second half of the usual sleep period (AASM 2005).

Nightmares are quite common among children and tend to decrease with age, but they can occur at any age. Having a history of trauma can increase the likelihood of having nightmares as an adult. People with acute stress disorder or post-traumatic stress disorder usually have frequent nightmares or flashbacks that involve reliving or replaying past traumas. (Acute stress disorder typically lasts between two and thirty days, whereas post-traumatic stress disorder lasts for more than one month.) Nightmares also occur more frequently among people with borderline personality disorder, schizoid personality disorder, and schizophrenia (Broughton 1999). In addition, some medications can cause increased nightmares, such as certain antidepressants, Parkinson's drugs, and drugs for high blood pressure (AASM 2005).

If you have nightmare disorder, supportive psychotherapy can be helpful, as can cognitive behavioral therapy. Reducing the amount of stress in your life and improving your skills for coping with stressful situations can also provide relief. It's also important not to deprive yourself of sleep and to practice good sleep hygiene. And although it may not always be possible, telling someone else about your nightmare upon awakening during the night may help you feel reassured and supported, and help you fall back asleep more easily.

SUMMING UP

This chapter discussed the most common parasomnias. As with other sleep disorders, it's important to seek help from a qualified professional if you think you may have one of these disorders. Although some are more problematic than others, any of them can affect your overall sleep quality and possibly even your daytime functioning. In addition, parasomnias can often be the result of another, underlying sleep disorder that causes arousals, such as restless legs syndrome, periodic limb movement disorder, or obstructive sleep apnea. For that reason, if you have one of the parsomnias discussed in this chapter, it would be a good idea to consult with a sleep specialist to determine whether you have an underlying sleep disorder.

CHAPTER 12

Women and Sleep

As I was writing this book, many people asked me if I was going to address sleep issues specific to women. Since women experience so many biological changes throughout the life span, it seemed appropriate to include a chapter on this topic. While the sleep program provided in this book is useful for both men and women in overcoming insomnia, it's worthwhile to consider some additional factors that affect how women sleep, either due to their physiology, or during different stages of life.

MENSTRUATION

Many women experience menstrual symptoms such as bloating, cramps, and discomfort, all of which can disrupt sleep. The severity of these symptoms, and therefore their potential impact on sleep, varies widely among women. In addition, some women may experience more disturbed sleep and increased sleepiness during the day during menstruation, independent of menstrual symptoms (Manber and Bootzin 1997). They may take longer to fall asleep and experience an increased number of awakenings during the night, decreased sleep efficiency, and poorer overall sleep quality. The sleep disturbance tends to be confined to certain days of the menstrual cycle, however, so it isn't advisable to take sedative-hypnotics to deal with sleep problems related to menstruation. This could make the situation worse, causing rebound insomnia when you stop taking sleeping medications. Instead, simply be aware that your sleep may be more disrupted during your menstrual cycle and remember, if you practice good sleep hygiene and don't allow yourself to become anxious about it, it probably won't turn into a long-term problem.

Premenstrual syndrome (PMS) can also impair sleep. It only makes sense that if you experience cramps, bloating, and significant discomfort before getting your period, it might make it harder to sleep. Your mood may be depressed, irritable, or down in the dumps. Although research on this topic varies, some studies have shown that women with PMS may have such changes in their sleep architecture as increased stage N2 sleep and decreased REM or slow-wave sleep (Baker et al. 2007). If you have

PMS, you may be more sensitive to waking up during the night because of pain, discomfort, or other symptoms. It's important to maintain good sleep hygiene during this time and, again, remember that this is a transient problem that will pass. Realizing that your sleep may be disrupted due to PMS will decrease your chances of becoming anxious about the situation. You may find that using different pillows (like body pillows) can help with aches and pains. Some people find ibuprofen (for example, Motrin and Advil) or naproxen (for example, Aleve and Synflex) helpful for alleviating cramps. A warm bath before bed may also be helpful.

SEXUAL ACTIVITY

While men are often tired and worn out after sex, women may have the opposite reaction. So while men may drift off to sleep quickly after sex, many women are wide awake. It's unclear whether the reason for women being more awake is psychological or physiological. Perhaps it's both. For most women, sexual intimacy is an emotional, as well as physical, connection. This means that after sex you may feel like talking or sharing your feelings. That's hard to do when your partner has already fallen asleep! In addition, you may feel physically alert and not yet ready for sleep. Rather than trying to force your partner to talk or becoming frustrated that you feel wide awake, try to think relaxing, calming thoughts and put yourself more in the mood for sleep. It may take ten or fifteen minutes, but perhaps your body and mind just need a little time to unwind after sex. If you find it very difficult to fall asleep after sex, what about trying different times of the day? Sex in the morning or earlier in the evening may work better for you.

PREGNANCY

Pregnancy is a time of many physiological changes, and many of them can affect your sleep. Due to increased levels of progesterone, you may experience gastrointestinal symptoms such as bloating, increased gas, and abdominal discomfort; your bowels may also be more sluggish. You may find that these symptoms get worse when you lie down to go to sleep at night. It's also common to urinate more frequently during pregnancy, and this can certainly disrupt your sleep. If you find yourself waking up several times per night to urinate, know that it's just par for the course during pregnancy. Decreasing your fluid intake for the hour or so before bedtime, however, may help decrease the number of visits to the bathroom at night. Just be sure you don't avoid liquids for much longer than that, as you don't want to become dehydrated.

Aside from the physical discomfort you may experience at different times during your pregnancy, which can make it harder for you to sleep, you may also feel anxious, preoccupied, or worried. All are normal reactions at this time, and all of them can impact your sleep. Even just being very excited about this time in your life can make it harder for you to sleep. Try to talk to family or friends about how you're feeling. Your emotional reactions to your pregnancy are probably quite similar to what others have been through, and you can find some support in knowing that you aren't alone in how you're feeling.

Fatigue and Daytime Sleepiness

It's common to feel fatigued or sleepy during pregnancy, especially during the first and last trimesters. In the beginning of pregnancy, increased levels of progesterone can make you feel sleepy. You may find yourself napping during the day even though you don't normally take naps. In addition, you've probably decreased or even stopped your intake of caffeine. That, coupled with increased progesterone, can make you feel more sleepy during the day. This doesn't usually last the entire pregnancy, but you can expect to feel quite sleepy for at least a few weeks during early pregnancy. This is totally normal.

Just be aware that if you're having trouble sleeping at night, napping can worsen that problem. If you desperately feel like you need to nap during the day, then your body clearly needs more rest. Because your body is going through so many changes, a nap may be an important way to rejuvenate yourself and feel better. But since it could be making your nighttime sleep worse, try to limit the length of your naps. Napping for thirty minutes or an hour will probably have less of an effect on your nighttime sleep than napping for two to three hours.

Discomfort and Pain

During pregnancy you may experience pain or discomfort at times. Lower back pain is quite common, especially later in pregnancy. In fact, lower back pain occurs in over 50 percent of all pregnancies (Kryger 2000). Joint and muscle pain may occur due to increased body weight. Any aches and pains can affect your sleep and keep you up at night. In fact, you may feel more pain when you're lying in bed at night than at other times. This is because you don't have any distractions when you're lying in bed at night. This isn't only true during pregnancy. Pain often worsens at night because you aren't actively engaging in other activities and as a result are more focused on the sensations in your body. Leg cramps are also quite common during pregnancy and can wake you up with considerable pain.

If it's difficult for you to find a comfortable position to sleep in, try using a pregnancy pillow, a body pillow, or various small pillows. If your lower back hurts, for example, you may be able to place a small pillow underneath it to help relieve some discomfort. After sixteen weeks of pregnancy, you shouldn't sleep on your back for the remainder of your pregnancy (Curtis and Schuler 2004). This is because the baby's weight can put pressure on your inferior vena cava, the main vein that transports blood from your lower body back to your heart. This can lower your blood pressure to unhealthy levels and also reduce blood flow to your baby. If you're used to sleeping on your back, it can be hard to get used to sleeping on your side. Try putting pillows or a wedge next to your back so you don't end up rolling over onto your back during the night while you're sleeping. Try not to feel frustrated if you can't seem to find a comfortable position. As time goes on, your body will adjust to your new sleeping position and the end result (your new baby) is certainly worth this temporary sacrifice.

Sciatica

Sciatic nerve pain can occur during pregnancy. If you've experienced this before, you know that it can be extremely painful. The pain typically starts in one buttock and goes down the back or side of one leg. Since the sciatic nerve is behind the uterus and runs down to the legs and feet, increased pressure from your growing baby may compress this nerve during pregnancy (Curtis and Schuler 2004). Sciatic nerve pain can also be caused by damage to the vertebrae or disks, like a slipped disk, which causes inflammation in the tissues around the nerve or even direct pressure on the nerve. You can try to relieve pain by lying on the opposite side. You may also get some relief from massage or certain exercises. A physical therapist may be able to advise you on the types of exercises to do, but always check with your doctor before seeking treatment.

Gastrointestinal Changes

Higher levels of progesterone in your body during pregnancy can lead to increased gas, bloating, and even burping. This is because progesterone relaxes smooth muscle tissues throughout your body, including the muscles in your gastrointestinal tract. Even in the early weeks of pregnancy, before you are showing, you may experience discomfort in your tummy, especially after eating heavier meals. You may benefit from eating smaller meals more often throughout the day rather than eating two or three large meals.

When you start getting bigger, your uterus takes up more space in your abdomen, which will slow digestion and make you feel bloated. You may also experience constipation or heartburn during pregnancy. All of these changes are normal during pregnancy, but they can still be quite annoying. Watching what you eat and cutting back on gas-promoting foods can be helpful—not just beans, but also broccoli, onions, cabbage, asparagus, and cauliflower. However, all of these foods are very healthful, so you wouldn't want to completely eliminate them from your diet; just cut down on them a bit, at least initially, and see how your body feels. Cutting out all carbonated beverages is always a good idea during pregnancy, as this can reduce gas and bloating. Exercise can also help your gut. It naturally helps to move things in the right direction and can make you feel better along the way.

Shortness of Breath and Respiratory Problems

Breathing is affected by pregnancy. You may experience shortness of breath during the day while walking or doing other types of exercise or activities that normally wouldn't cause this. The same is true at night. Pregnancy can make you snore even if that's unusual for you. In one study, 23 percent of women snored nightly at the end of the pregnancy, even though only 4 percent of them snored before they were pregnant (Kryger 2000). In this study, snorers were more likely to develop hypertension or preeclampsia. In addition, it was more likely that their developing babies were significantly below average weight, and their newborns were more likely to have lower Apgar scores—a measure that assesses the newborn's health immediately after birth. For these reasons, you may want to discuss over-the-counter treatment for snoring, such as nasal dilation, with your obstetrician. The risk of complications such as pulmonary hypertension, gestational diabetes mellitus, and preeclampsia is even higher if you have obstructive sleep apnea during pregnancy (Edwards et al. 2002). If you think that you may have obstructive sleep apnea, it's crucial that you get immediate treatment with continuous positive airway pressure (CPAP); otherwise, your health and your infant's health could be compromised.

To decrease snoring and other respiratory disturbances during sleep, avoid sleeping on your back. This is true for all snorers, not just pregnant women. As mentioned earlier, this is especially important after sixteen weeks of pregnancy, but if you notice yourself snoring earlier in your pregnancy or feeling short of breath, you may do better sleeping on your side.

Restless Legs Syndrome

If you start to experience a creepy-crawly sensation in your legs at night during your pregnancy, like an uncomfortable tingling feeling that makes you want to move your legs, you're not alone. In one study, researchers found that nearly 20 percent of pregnant women had restless legs syndrome (RLS), which is greater than the prevalence of RLS in the general population (Suzuki et al. 2003). This may be due to iron deficiency, as your body requires more iron during pregnancy (Cotter and O'Keeffe 2006), or endocrine changes that occur during pregnancy (Winkelmann et al. 2000). The symptoms often go away on their own after delivery (Goodman, Brodie, and Ayida 1988), but there are a few things you can do to improve the symptoms while you have them.

Nonpharmacological steps you can take to improve your symptoms of RLS include moderate daily exercise emphasizing the legs, stretching (particularly the legs) prior to bedtime, and avoiding caffeine, nicotine, and alcohol. It's also important to rule out an underlying vitamin or mineral deficiency, so ask your doctor to check your levels of iron, ferritin, magnesium, vitamin B$_{12}$, and folate (Montplaisir et al. 2000). Sometimes supplementing the vitamins or minerals you're deficient in can resolve symptoms of RLS. Of course, you should check with your obstetrician first before starting to take any new supplements during pregnancy.

Nocturnal Leg Cramps

While RLS usually causes trouble falling asleep, nocturnal leg cramps due to sudden tightening of the muscles in your legs can wake you up during the night. It's estimated that leg cramps occur in 5 to 30 percent of pregnant women (Dahle et al. 1995). The cramps occur suddenly during your sleep, leaving you awake and in pain in your bed. Standing for long periods of time during the day or sitting with your legs crossed can worsen this problem.

Studies have shown that magnesium supplements can help with pregnancy-related leg cramps (Dahle et al. 1995). You should, however, ask your doctor before taking any new supplements. You may find it helpful to stretch your calf muscles during the day and before bedtime and rotate your ankles or wiggle your toes while you're sitting. As with RLS, exercising the legs daily may help, so try taking a walk each day. Because dehydration can cause your muscles to cramp, make sure you drink plenty of water each day.

If you get a leg cramp during the night, don't point your toes! This can make the cramp worse. Instead, straighten your leg, heel first, and slowly flex your toes back toward your shins. This will decrease the muscle spasm, and eventually the pain will disappear. You can also try massaging your leg or walking around for a few minutes. These techniques should make the pain go away. If you have more persistent, chronic pain, tenderness, or swelling in your legs, be sure to tell your doctor immediately. Blood clots can occur during pregnancy, and they require immediate treatment.

THE SECOND SHIFT

Although many men are playing a much bigger role in child care and sharing household responsibilities with their wives, many of the more traditional duties of looking after the house and the children still fall on the shoulders of women. Authors Arlie Russell Hochschild and Anne Machung (2003) coined the phrase "the second shift" to describe what often occurs when working women get home from their jobs each evening: They begin a second shift of cooking, cleaning, looking after their children, and so on. There's no doubt that having significant responsibilities at home each evening can lead to increased stress and anxiety in your life. It can be hard for working mothers to find the necessary balance of work and play in their lives when they come home to a set of chores and responsibilities. This is not to say that men don't also experience additional responsibilities when they get home from work, but society often frowns upon mothers who don't seem to be able to juggle their career and home life without any complaints. After a hard day at work, it can be frustrating and overwhelming to come home to a list of things to do, but it is a common occurrence that can cause stress for many women. This stress can, undoubtedly, cause difficulties sleeping at night. If you don't have time to relax when you get home, it can be tough to wind down and get your mind into a relaxed state when it's bedtime. If you feel that your sleep is affected by all of the pressures of being a working mother, try to seek support from your spouse, other family members, and friends. Give yourself a break and know that no one is perfect. Even if it means picking up dinner on the way home from work once a week rather than cooking yourself, the time and stress you'll save yourself doing so could be just what you need.

PERIMENOPAUSE AND MENOPAUSE

You may start to experience sleep problems during perimenopause or menopause. At this time, your body produces less estrogen and progesterone. According to research, about 24 percent of premenopausal women say they have trouble sleeping, compared with 35 percent of perimenopausal and 41 percent of postmenopausal women (Alexander et al. 2007). These sleeping problems may be due, at least in part, to hot flashes or night sweats, which can make it hard to fall asleep and can also cause more awakenings during the night. Dressing in lighter clothes and making sure that the bedroom is a comfortable temperature may help decrease hot flashes or night sweats. For some women, perimenopause and menopause can cause sleep disruption due to increased trips to the bathroom at night. Menopausal women may also be at increased risk of sleep-disordered breathing and snoring, thus causing more disrupted sleep (Badheka, Sameen, and Rozensky 2005). In addition to difficulty sleeping, you may experience decreased energy and more fatigue during the day. This is likely due to sleeping poorly, since fragmented sleep at night can cause daytime sleepiness and fatigue. And just like insomnia occurring at other stages of life and among men, insomnia during perimenopause and menopause is associated with a higher incidence of anxiety and depression.

Cognitive behavioral therapy can be useful in overcoming sleep problems that occur during perimenopause and menopause (Alexander et al. 2007). This approach includes techniques discussed in this workbook, like improved sleep hygiene, relaxation exercises, stimulus control, sleep restriction, and managing stress and anxiety. The cognitive component of the sleep program can be particularly helpful in overcoming fears you may have developed, like the possible consequences of decreased sleep that you may have catastrophized in your head.

Some women find relief in hormone replacement therapy. That is an issue you should discuss with your doctor, carefully weighing the benefits and risks, to see if it's the right choice for you. Some studies have shown that estrogen replacement therapy can improve the quality of a woman's sleep, while other studies have found no differences (Bliwise 2000). For that reason, it's unclear if hormone replacement therapy will truly improve your sleep, and it may vary from woman to woman.

SUMMING UP

Insomnia is more common in women than in men. The reasons for this vary from person to person, but hormonal changes and physiological factors like menstruation and pregnancy definitely contribute to this phenomenon. By using the methods described in this book, such as learning to decrease your daytime stress, improving your sleep hygiene, and taking time for relaxation, you can improve the overall quality of your sleep.

Resources

USEFUL WEBSITES

National Sleep Foundation (NSF)
 www.sleepfoundation.org
The NSF is a nonprofit organization supporting education, research, and advocacy related to sleep disorders. The site provides information on sleep disorders, sleep hygiene, and other sleep-related issues. It's useful for both the public and sleep professionals.

American Insomnia Association (AIA)
 www.americaninsomniaassociation.org
This patient-based organization promotes and advocates education, research, and awareness about insomnia in order to help people with insomnia. Its website provides information on insomnia, its causes, treatment options, and medications, and additional resources on finding a sleep center or qualified insomnia specialist.

American Psychological Association (APA)
 www.apa.org
This site for both psychologists and the public has information on mental illness. You can find useful information on sleep, depression, anxiety, and other topics in the "Psychology Topics" section. If you're looking for a psychologist in your area, click on the quick link "Find a Psychologist" for a list of psychologists across the country who are members of the APA.

American Academy of Sleep Medicine (AASM)
www.aasmnet.org
To find an accredited sleep laboratory in your area, click on the link "Patients & Public" and then "Find a Sleep Center" for a listing of locations by state. An overnight sleep study can be very helpful if you think you may have obstructive sleep apnea, periodic limb movement disorder, narcolepsy, or REM sleep behavior disorder.

Anxiety Disorders Association of America (ADAA)
www.adaa.org
This site provides information on anxiety disorders, their symptoms, and treatment, as well as a listing of support groups and professionals with expertise in anxiety disorders, and suggestions on ways to get help.

National Alliance on Mental Illness (NAMI)
www.nami.org
NAMI is a grassroots, self-help, nonprofit advocacy organization. Its website provides information on mental illness, resources in your community, and ways to learn more about mental disorders.

RELAXATION EXERCISES

A wide variety of relaxation exercises are available on CD and as MP3 downloads. Here are a few recommended resources for prerecorded relaxation exercises.

Stephanie A. Silberman, Ph.D., DABSM
For downloads of various relaxation exercises, you can visit my website at www.sleeppsychology.com and click on the relaxation exercises section.

Matthew McKay, Ph.D., and Patrick Fanning
The Relaxation and Stress Reduction Audio Series (available from New Harbinger Publications and Amazon.com)

Applied Relaxation Training, ISBN: 978-1-57224-6379

Meditation and Autogenics, ISBN: 978-1-57224-6409

Body Awareness and Imagination, ISBN: 978-1-57224-6386

Progressive Relaxation and Breathing, ISBN: 978-1-57224-6393

Stress Reduction, ISBN: 978-1-57224-6416, Audio CD

The Daily Relaxer Audio Companion: Soothing Guided Meditations for Deep Relaxation Anytime, Anywhere: ISBN: 978-1-57224-6362, Double set audio CD

Scott Gauthier
Welcome to Earth: Explorations in Body Awareness and Relaxation. In particular, the Deep Relaxation exercise is similar to the relaxation exercises in this workbook. The CD is available at Amazon.com and CDbaby.com. For downloads, you can go to iTunes or Rhapsody.

References

Alexander, J. L., T. Neylan, K. Kotz, L. Dennerstein, G. Richardson, and R. Rosenbaum. 2007. Assessment and treatment for insomnia and fatigue in the symptomatic menopausal woman with psychiatric comorbidity. *Expert Review of Neurotherapeutics* 7(11 suppl.):S139-S155.

American Academy of Sleep Medicine (AASM). 2005. *International Classification of Sleep Disorders: Diagnostic and Coding Manual.* 2nd edition. Westchester, IL: American Academy of Sleep Medicine.

American Psychiatric Association. 1994. *Diagnostic and Statistical Manual of Mental Disorders.* 4th edition. Washington, DC: American Psychiatric Association.

Atkins, W. 2008. Got sleep? CDC says 1 out of 10 Americans are sleep deprived! www.itwire.com/content/view/16931/1066/. Accessed August 15, 2008.

Badheka, N. H., M. T. Sameen, and R. Rozensky. 2005. Managing menopause and sleep. *Sleep Review,* September-October.

Baker, F. C., T. L. Kahan, J. Trinder, and I. M. Colrain. 2007. Sleep quality and the sleep electroencephalogram in women with severe premenstrual syndrome. *Sleep* 30(10):1283-1291.

Basner, R. C. 2005. Shift-work sleep disorder: The glass is more than half empty. *New England Journal of Medicine* 353(5):519-521.

Belleville, G., and C. M. Morin. 2008. Hypnotic discontinuation in chronic insomnia: Impact of psychological distress, readiness to change, and self-efficacy. *Health Psychology* 27(2):239-248.

Benca, R. 2000. Mood disorders. In *Principles and Practice of Sleep Medicine,* 3rd edition, edited by M. H. Kryger, T. Roth, and W. C. Dement. Philadelphia: W. B. Saunders Company.

Berg, D. 2008. Biomarkers for the early detection of Parkinson's and Alzheimer's disease. *Neurodegenerative Diseases* 5(3-4):133-136.

Bliwise, D. L. 2000. Normal aging. In *Principles and Practice of Sleep Medicine*, 3rd edition, edited by M. H. Kryger, T. Roth, and W. C. Dement. Philadelphia: W. B. Saunders Company.

Bliwise, D. L., and F. P. Ansari. 2007. Insomnia associated with valerian and melatonin usage in the 2002 National Health Interview Survey. *Sleep* 30(7):881-884.

Boon, H. S., and A. H. C. Wong. 2003. Kava: A test case for Canada's new approach to natural health products. *Canadian Medical Association Journal* 169(11):1163-1164.

Bootzin, R. R. 1972. Stimulus control treatment for insomnia. *Proceedings of the 80th Annual Convention of the American Psychological Association* 7:395-396.

Bootzin, R. R., and S. P. Rider. 2000. Behavioral techniques and biofeedback for insomnia. In *Understanding Sleep: The Evaluation and Treatment of Sleep Disorders*, edited by M. R. Pressman and W. C. Orr. Washington, DC: American Psychological Association.

Bourne, E. J. 2005. *The Anxiety and Phobia Workbook.* 4th edition. Oakland, CA: New Harbinger Publications.

Bowman, T. J., and V. Mohsenin. 2003. Synopsis of sleep. In *Review of Sleep Medicine*, edited by T. J. Bowman. Amsterdam: Butterworth Heinemann.

Brielmaier, B. D. 2006. Eszopiclone (Lunesta): A new nonbenzodiazepine hypnotic agent. *Proceedings (Baylor University Medical Center)* 19(1):54-59.

Broughton, R. J. 1999. Behavioral parasomnias. In *Sleep Disorders Medicine: Basic Science, Technical Consideration, and Clinical Aspects*, 2nd edition, edited by S. Chokroverty. Boston: Butterworth-Heinemann.

Cagnacci, A., S. Arangino, A. Renzi, A. M. Paoletti, G. B. Melis, P. Cagnacci, and A. Volpe. 2001. Influence of melatonin administration on glucose tolerance and insulin sensitivity of postmenopausal women. *Clinical Endocrinology (Oxford)* 54(3):339-346.

Cappuccio, F. P., S. Stranges, N. B. Kandala, M. A. Miller, F. M. Taggart, M. Kumari, J. E. Ferrie, M. J. Shipley, E. J. Brunner, and M. G. Marmot. 2007. Gender-specific associations of short sleep duration with prevalent and incident hypertension: The Whitehall II Study. *Hypertension* 50(4):693-700.

Carlson, N. R. 1998. *Physiology of Behavior.* 6th edition. Boston: Allyn and Bacon.

Chesson, Jr., A. L., W. M. Anderson, M. Littner, D. Davila, K. Hartse, S. Johnson, M. Wise, and J. Rafecas. 1999. Practice parameters for the nonpharmacological treatment of chronic insomnia: An American Academy of Sleep Medicine report. *Sleep* 22(8):1128-1133.

Cimolai, N. 2007. Zopiclone: Is it a pharmacologic agent for abuse? *Canadian Family Physician* 53(12):2124-2129.

Copinschi, G. 2005. Metabolic and endocrine effects of sleep deprivation. *Essential Psychopharmacology* 6(6):341-347.

Cotter, P. E., and S. T. O'Keeffe. 2006. Restless legs syndrome: Is it a real problem? *Therapeutics and Clinical Risk Management* 2(4):465-475.

Crispim, C. A., I. Zalcman, M. Dattilo, H. G. Padilha, S. Tufik, and M. T. de Mello. 2007. Relation between sleep and obesity: A literature review. [Article in Portuguese.] *Arquivos Brasileiros de Endocrinologia e Metabologia* 51(7):1041-1049.

Curcio, G., M. Ferrara, and L. De Gennaro. 2006. Sleep loss, learning capacity and academic performance. *Sleep Medicine Reviews* 10(5):323-337.

Curtis, G. B., and J. Schuler. 2004. *Your Pregnancy Week: Week by Week.* 5th edition. Cambridge, MA: Da Capo Press.

Dahle, L. O., G. Berg, M. Hammar, M. Hurtig, and L. Larsson. 1995. The effect of oral magnesium substitution on pregnancy-induced leg cramps. *American Journal of Obstetrics and Gynecology* 173(1):175-180.

Edinger, J. D., M. K. Means, C. E. Carney, and A. D. Krystal. 2008. Psychomotor performance deficits and their relation to prior nights' sleep among individuals with primary insomnia. *Sleep* 31(5):599-607.

Edwards, N., P. G. Middleton, D. M. Blyton, and C. E. Sullivan. 2002. Sleep disordered breathing and pregnancy. *Thorax* 57(6):555-558.

Fennell, M. J. V. 1998. Depression. In *Cognitive Behaviour Therapy for Psychiatric Problems: A Practical Guide,* edited by K. Hawton, P. M. Salkovskis, J. Kirk, and D. M. Clark. Oxford, England: Oxford University Press.

Foley, D. J., A. A. Monjan, S. L. Brown, E. M. Simonsick, R. B. Wallace, and D. G. Blazer. 1995. Sleep complaints among elderly persons: An epidemiologic study of three communities. *Sleep* 18(6):425-432.

Fu, P. P., Q. Xia, L. Guo, H. Yu, and P. C. Chan. 2008. Toxicity of kava kava. *Journal of Environmental Science and Health. Part C, Environmental Carcinogensis and Ecotoxicology Reviews* 26(1):89-112.

Gangwisch, J. E., S. B. Heymsfield, B. Boden-Albala, R. M. Buijs, F. Kreier, T. G. Pickering, A. G. Rundle, G. K. Zammit, and D. Malaspina. 2006. Short sleep duration as a risk factor for hypertension: Analyses of the first National Health and Nutrition Examination Survey. *Hypertension* 47(5):833-839.

Gangwisch, J. E., D. Malaspina, B. Boden-Albala, and S. B. Heymsfield. 2005. Inadequate sleep as a risk factor for obesity: Analyses of the NHANES I. *Sleep* 28(10):1217-1220.

Gardner, D. M., R. J. Baldessarini, and P. Waraich. 2005. Modern antipsychotic drugs: A critical overview. *Canadian Medical Association Journal* 172(13):1703-1711.

Gibson, E. S., A. C. Powles, L. Thabane, S. O'Brien, D. S. Molnar, N. Trajanovic, R. Ogilvie, C. Shapiro, M. Yan, and L. Chilcott-Tanser. 2006. "Sleepiness" is serious in adolescence: Two surveys of 3235 Canadian students. *BMC Public Health* 6:116.

Gillin, J. C., and S. P. A. Drummond. 2000. Medication and substance abuse. In *Principles and Practice of Sleep Medicine,* 3rd edition, edited by M. H. Kryger, T. Roth, and W. C. Dement. Philadelphia: W. B. Saunders Company.

Glass, J., K. L. Lanctot, N. Herrmann, B. A. Sproule, and U. E. Busto. 2005. Sedative hypnotics in older people with insomnia: Meta-analysis of risks and benefits. *BMJ* 331(7256):1169-1175.

Glotzbach, S. F., and H. C. Heller. 2000. Temperature regulation. In *Principles and Practice of Sleep Medicine*, 3rd edition, edited by M. H. Kryger, T. Roth, and W. C. Dement. Philadelphia: W. B. Saunders Company.

Goodman, J. D. S., C. Brodie, and G. A. Ayida. 1988. Restless leg syndrome in pregnancy. *BMJ* 297(6656):1101-1102.

Grigg-Damberger, M. 2006. Why a polysomnogram should become part of the diagnostic evaluation of stroke and transient ischemic attack. *Journal of Clinical Neurophysiology* 23(1):21-38.

Guardiola-Lemaitre, B. 1997. Toxicology of melatonin. *Journal of Biological Rhythms* 12(6):697-706.

Hassed, C. 2001. How humour keeps you well. *Australian Family Physician* 30(1):25-28.

Hauri, P. J. 1998. Insomnia. *Clinics in Chest Medicine* 19(1):157-168.

Hindmarch, I., E. Legangneux, N. Stanley, S. Emegbo, and J. Dawson. 2006. A double-blind, placebo-controlled investigation of the residual psychomotor and cognitive effects of zolpidem-MR in healthy elderly volunteers. *British Journal of Clinical Pharmacology* 62(5):538-545.

Hochschild, A. R., and A. Machung. 2003. *The Second Shift*. New York: Penguin Books.

Holbrook, A. M. 2004. Treating insomnia: Use of drugs is rising despite evidence of harm and little meaningful benefit. *BMJ* 329(7476):1198-1199.

Iber, C, S. Ancoli-Israel, A. Chesson, and S. F. Quan. 2007. *The AASM Manual for the Scoring of Sleep and Associated Events: Rules, Terminology and Technical Specifications*. Westchester, IL: American Academy of Sleep Medicine.

Irwin, M. R., M. Wang, D. Ribeiro, H. J. Cho, R. Olmstead, E. C. Breen, O. Martinez-Maza, and S. Cole. 2008. Sleep loss activates cellular inflammatory signaling. *Biological Psychiatry* 64(6):538-540.

Johns, M. W. 1991. A new method for measuring daytime sleepiness: The Epworth Sleepiness Scale. *Sleep* 14(6):540-545.

Kahol, K., M. J. Leyba, M. Deka, V. Deka, S. Mayes, M. Smith, J. J. Ferrara, and S. Panchanathan. 2008. Effect of fatigue on psychomotor and cognitive and skills. *American Journal of Surgery* 195(2):195-204.

Kato, K., K. Hirai, K. Nishiyama, O. Uchikawa, K. Fukatsu, S. Ohkawa, Y. Kawamata, S. Hinuma, and M. Miyamoto. 2005. Neurochemical properties of ramelteon (TAK-375), a selective MT1/MT2 receptor agonist. *Neuropharmacology* 48(2):301-310.

Kemper, K. J., and S. Shannon. 2007. CAM therapies to promote healthy moods. *Pediatric Clinics of North America* 54(6):901-924.

Knutson, K. L., K. Spiegel, P. Penev, and E. V. Cauter. 2007. The metabolic consequences of sleep deprivation. *Sleep Medicine Reviews* 11(3):168-178.

Kryger, M. H. 2000. Restrictive lung disorders. In *Principles and Practice of Sleep Medicine*, 3rd edition, edited by M. H. Kryger, T. Roth, and W. C. Dement. Philadelphia: W. B. Saunders Company.

Kuhn, B. R. 2001. Pediatric parasomnias. *Sleep Review*, spring issue, 29-32.

Landolt, H. P., E. Werth, A. A. Borberly, and D. J. Dijk. 1995. Caffeine intake (200 mg) in the morning affects human sleep and EEG power spectra at night. *Brain Research* 675(1-2):67-74.

Leipzig, R. M., R. G. Cumming, and M. E. Tinetti. 1999. Drugs and falls in older people: A systematic review and meta-analysis: I. Psychotropic drugs. *Journal of the American Geriatric Society* 47(1):30-39.

Leppämäki, S., J. Haukka, J. Lönnqvist, and T. Partonen. 2004. Drop-out and mood improvement: A randomized controlled trial with light exposure and physical exercise. *BMC Psychiatry* 4:22-32

Lieberman, J. A. 2007. Update on the safety considerations in the management of insomnia with hypnotics: Incorporating modified-release formulations into primary care. *Primary Care Companion to the Journal of Clinical Psychiatry* 9(1):25-31.

Lude, S., M. Torok, S. Dieterle, R. Jaggi, K. B. Buter, and S. Krahenbuhl. 2008. Hepatocellular toxicity of kava leaf and root extracts. *Phytomedicine* 16(1-2):120-131.

Lusardi, P., E. Piazza, and R. Fogari. 2000. Cardiovascular effects of melatonin in hypertensive patients well controlled by nifedipine: A 24-hour study. *British Journal of Clinical Pharmacology* 49(5):423-427.

Magee, E. 2004. 7 ways to de-stress your diet: Nutritional tricks to help you stave off stress. www.webmd.com/diet/features/7-ways-to-de-stree-your-diet. Accessed August 14, 2008.

Mai, E., and D. J. Buysse. 2008. Insomnia: Prevalence, impact, pathogenesis, differential diagnosis, and evaluation. *Sleep Medicine Clinics* 3(2):167-174.

Manber, R., and R. R. Bootzin. 1997. Sleep and the menstrual cycle. *Health Psychology* 16(3):209-214.

McCall, W. V. 2004. Sleep in the elderly: Burden, diagnosis, and treatment. *Primary Care Companion to the Journal of Clinical Psychiatry* 6(1):9-20.

McCall, W. V., A. B. Fleischer, and S. R. Feldman. 2001. Diagnostic codes associated with hypnotic medications during outpatient physician-patient encounters in the United States from 1990-1998. *Sleep* 25(2):221-223.

Mendelson, W. B. 2000. Hypnotics: Basic mechanisms and pharmacology. In *Principles and Practice of Sleep Medicine*, 3rd edition, edited by M. H. Kryger, T. Roth, and W. C. Dement. Philadelphia: W. B. Saunders Company.

Millar, K., A. J. Asbury, A. W. Bowman, M. T. Hosey, K. Martin, T. Musiello, and R. R. Welbury. 2007. A randomized placebo-controlled trial of the effects of midazolam premedication on children's postoperative cognition. *Anaesthesia* 62(9):923-930.

Mills, E., R. Singh, C. Ross, E. Ernst, and K. Wilson. 2004. Impact of federal safety advisories on health food store advice. *Journal of General Internal Medicine* 19(3):269-272.

Montplaisir, J., A. Nicolas, R. Godbout, and A. Walters. 2000. Restless legs syndrome and periodic limb movement disorder. In *Principles and Practice of Sleep Medicine*, 3rd edition, edited by M. H. Kryger, T. Roth, and W. C. Dement. Philadelphia: W. B. Saunders Company.

Morgenthaler, T., M. Kramer, C. Alessi, L. Friedman, B. Boehlecke, T. Brown, J. Coleman, V. Kapur, T. Lee-Chiong, J. Owens, J. Pancer, and T. Swick. 2006. Practice parameters for the psychological and behavioral treatment of insomnia: An update. An American Academy of Sleep Medicine report. *Sleep* 29(11):1415-1419.

Morgenthaler, T. I., and M. H. Silber. 2002. Amnestic sleep-related eating disorder associated with zolpidem. *Sleep Medicine* 3(4):323-327.

Morin, C. M. 1993. *Insomnia: Psychological Assessment and Management.* New York: Guilford Press.

Morin, C. M., R. R. Bootzin, D. J. Buysse, J. D. Edinger, C. A. Espie, and K. L. Lichstein. 2006. Psychological and behavioral treatment of insomnia: Update of the recent evidence (1998-2004). *Sleep* 29(11):1398-1414.

Morin, C. M., C. Colecchi, J. Stone, R. Sood, and D. Brink. 1999. Behavioral and pharmacological therapies for late-life insomnia. *The Journal of the American Medical Association* 281(11):991-999.

Morin, C. M., P. J. Hauri, C. A. Espie, A. J. Spielman, D. J. Buysse, and R. R. Bootzin. 1999. Nonpharmacological treatment of chronic insomnia. An American Academy of Sleep Medicine review. *Sleep* 22(8):1134-1156.

Najjar, M. 2007. Zolpidem and amnestic sleep related eating disorder. *Journal of Clinical Sleep Medicine* 3(6):637-638.

National Institutes of Health. 2005. NIH state-of-the-science conference statement on manifestations and management of chronic insomnia in adults. *NIH Consensus Science Statements* 22(2):1-30.

National Sleep Foundation. 2002. *Sleep in America* poll prepared by WB&A Market Research. Washington, DC: National Sleep Foundation.

National Sleep Foundation. 2007. *Sleep in America* poll prepared by WB&A Market Research. Washington, DC: National Sleep Foundation.

Neubauer, D. N. 2007. The evolution and development of insomnia pharmacotherapies. *Journal of Clinical Sleep Medicine* 3(5 suppl.):S11-S15.

Ohayon, M. 2002. Epidemiology of insomnia: what we know and what we still need to learn. *Sleep Medicine Reviews* 6(2):97-111.

Park, L. T., J. D. Matthews, G. Maytal, and T. A. Stern. 2007. Evaluation and treatment of poor sleep. *Primary Care Companion to the Journal of Clinical Psychiatry* 9(3):224-229.

Poppen, R. 1998. *Behavioral Relaxation Training and Assessment.* 2nd edition. Thousand Oaks, CA: Sage Publications.

Ray, O., and C. Ksir. 1993. *Drugs, Society, and Human Behavior.* 6th edition. St. Louis, MO: Mosby.

Richardson, G. S. 2007. Human physiological models of insomnia. *Sleep Medicine* 8(4 suppl.):S9-S14.

Roehrs, T., F. J. Zorick, and T. Roth. 2000. Transient and short-term insomnias. In *Principles and Practice of Sleep Medicine*, 3rd edition, edited by M. H. Kryger, T. Roth, and W. C. Dement. Philadelphia: W. B. Saunders Company.

Rothenberg, S. A. 2000. Introduction to sleep disorders. In *Understanding Sleep: The Evaluation and Treatment of Sleep Disorders*, edited by M. R. Pressman and W. C. Orr. Washington, DC: American Psychological Association.

Sateia, M. J., K. Doghramji, P. J. Hauri, and C. M. Morin. 2000. Evaluation of chronic insomnia. *Sleep* 23(2):1-65.

Schenck, C. H., and M. W. Mahowald. 2003. REM sleep behavior disorder. In *Sleep and Movement Disorders*, edited by S. Chokroverty, W. A. Hening, and A. S. Walters. Philadelphia: Butterworth-Heinemann.

Schilit, R., and E. S. Lisansky Gomberg. 1991. *Drugs and Behavior.* Newbury Park, CA: Sage Publications.

Sherwood, L. 2006. *Fundamentals of Physiology: A Human Perspective.* 3rd edition. Belmont, CA: Thomson Brooks/Cole Publishing.

Shimazaki, M., and J. L. Martin. 2007. Do herbal agents have a place in the treatment of sleep problems in long-term care? *Journal of the American Medical Directors Association* 8(4):248-252.

Simon, G. E., and E. J. Ludman. 2006. Outcome of new benzodiazepine prescriptions to older adults in primary care. *General Hospital Psychiatry* 28(5):374-378.

Spielman, A. J., and M. W. Anderson. 1999. The clinical interview and treatment planning as a guide to understanding the nature of insomnia: The CCNY insomnia interview. In *Sleep Disorders Medicine: Basic Science, Technical Considerations, and Clinical Aspects*, 2nd edition, edited by S. Chokroverty. Boston: Butterworth-Heinemann.

Spielman, A. J., P. Saskin, and M. J. Thorpy. 1987. Treatment of chronic insomnia by restriction of time in bed. *Sleep* 10(1):45-56.

Stoller, M. K. 1994. Economic effects of insomnia. *Clinical Therapeutics* 16(5):873-897.

Suzuki, K., T. Ohida, T. Sone, S. Takemura, E. Yokoyama, T. Miyake, S. Harano, S. Motojima, M. Suga, and E. Ibuka. 2003. The prevalence of restless legs syndrome among pregnant women in Japan and the relationship between restless legs syndrome and sleep problems. *Sleep* 26(6):673-677.

Vandewalle, G., B. Middleton, S. M. Rajaratnam, B. M. Stone, B. Thorleifsdottir, J. Arendt, and D. J. Dijk. 2007. Robust circadian rhythm in heart rate and its variability: Influence of exogenous melatonin and photoperiod. *Journal of Sleep Research* 16(2):148-155.

Walsh, J. K., and C. L. Engelhardt. 1999. The direct economic costs of insomnia in the United States for 1995. *Sleep* 22(2 suppl.):S386-S393.

Weaver, D. R. 1997. Reproductive safety of melatonin: A "wonder drug" to wonder about. *Journal of Biological Rhythms* 12(6):707-708.

Winkelmann, J., T. C. Wetter, V. Collado-Seidel, T. Gasser, M. Dichgans, A. Yassouridis, and C. Trenkwalder. 2000. Clinical characteristics and frequency of the hereditary restless legs syndrome in a population of 200 patients. *Sleep* 23(5):1-6.

Wooltorton, E. 2002a. Brief safety updates: Acetaminophen, ASA, and kava. *Canadian Medical Association Journal* 167(9):1034.

Wooltorton, E. 2002b. Herbal kava: Reports of liver toxicity. *Canadian Medical Association Journal* 166(6):777.

Zammit, G., M. Erman, S. Wang-Weigand, S. Sainati, J. Zhang, and T. Roth. 2007. Evaluation of the efficacy and safety of ramelteon in subjects with chronic insomnia. *Journal of Clinical Sleep Medicine* 3(5):495-504.

Stephanie A. Silberman, Ph.D., DABSM, is a clinical psychologist who specializes in using cognitive behavioral therapy for the treatment of sleep disorders, depression, and anxiety. She is a consultant for many sleep laboratories and maintains a private practice in the Fort Lauderdale, FL, area.

Foreword writer **Charles M. Morin, Ph.D.,** is professor of psychology and director of the Sleep Research Center at the Université Laval in Quebec City. He holds a Canada Research Chair on Sleep Disorders and is past president of the Canadian Sleep Society. Morin is associate editor for the journals *Sleep* and *Behavioral Sleep Medicine.* He has published four books and more than 150 articles and chapters.

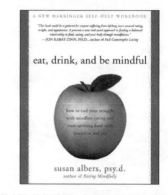
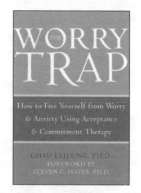
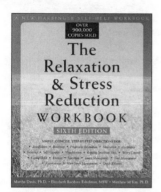
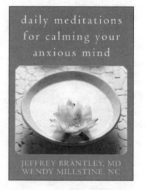
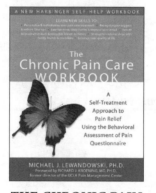
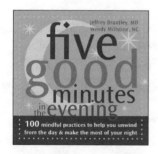
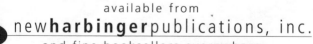